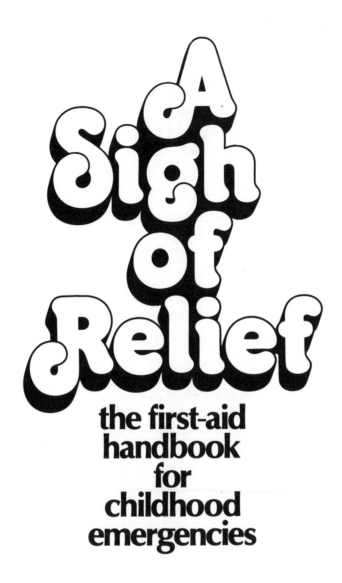

A Sigh of Relief

the first-aid handbook for childhood emergencies

Produced by Martin I. Green

BANTAM BOOKS
TORONTO • NEW YORK • LONDON

the first-aid handbook for childhood emergencies

A Bantam Book / September 1977

Library of Congress Catalog Card Number: 77-81392
ISBN 0-553-01155-3

Published simultaneously in the United States and Canada

Bantam Books are published by Bantam Books, Inc. Its trademark, consisting of the
words "Bantam Books" and the portrayal of a bantam, is registered in the United States
Patent Office and in other countries. Marca Registrada. Bantam Books, Inc., 666 Fifth
Avenue, New York, New York 10019.

Printed In The United States Of America
0 9 8 7 6 5 4

We wish to thank the following for providing us with information, for making their facilities and staff available to us, and for reviewing and commenting on the manuscript during its various phases.

American National Red Cross
Washington, D.C.

Boston Children's Medical Center
Boston, Massachusetts

National Clearinghouse For Poison Control Centers
Department Of Health, Education And Welfare
Bethesda, Maryland

National Safety Council
Chicago, Illinois

We would also like to thank the American Academy Of Pediatrics and the U.S. Consumer Product Safety Commission for information provided.

Credits

Produced By
Martin I. Green

Edited By
Ross Firestone

Research Director
Paul A. Cirincione

Illustrated By
Bobbi Bongard

Designed By
Bobbi Bongard & Martin I. Green

Assistant Designer
Mary Sipp Green

Research Associate
Mary Sipp Green

Medical Consultant
Kenneth Jay Solomon, M.D.

Editorial Assistant
Bernice Cirincione

Mechanical Art By
Sipp Graphic Design Studio

Special thanks to Seymour Z. Baum, Frank Bongard, Alan Douglas, Gail Firestone, Steve Futterman, Robert Goldoff, Lee Goldstein, Robert Moses, Harvey Rottenberg, Service Art Studio and Typographic Concepts.

Berkshire Studio
PRODUCTION
West Stockbridge, Massachusetts 01266

FOR
MY MOTHER AND FATHER,
MARY,
OUR SON JARED
AND
ALL CHILDREN EVERYWHERE.

Contents

Preface

By Vincent L. Tofany
President, National Safety Council

A Sigh Of Relief is an interesting contribution to the literature on child safety. I hope it will be carefully read and widely used.

The book is divided into two parts. The first deals with the prevention of childhood accidents and the second with the action required after an accident has taken place. Prevention is, of course, the single most important element in child safety. When successful, it makes emergency measures unnecessary.

There are few mysteries in accident prevention. The preparations, practices and required actions are usually, if not always, simple, obvious and based upon common sense. But as many writers have pointed out, common sense is an uncommon commodity and the obvious is often overlooked, so it is always useful to have these basic preventive measures brought to our attention.

And sometimes common sense is not enough. In the more than 60 years that the organized voluntary safety movement has been in existence in the United States, it has developed and tested a great variety of preventive techniques applicable to all ages and activities. The authors of this book have made extensive use of this body of work as collated and disseminated by the clearing house for safety information, the National Safety Council.

As every safety worker knows, no matter how ardently prevention may be advocated, there will always be failures in prevention which will lead to accidental injuries. It is entirely appropriate, then, that the second part of **A Sigh Of Relief** goes on to treat emergency management—"first aid" is perhaps the better known term. The emergency management section of this book has an original and, I believe, useful format designed to supply parents and other responsible adults with the needed information in quickly retrievable, highly graphic form.

Without question, parents who take seriously what they read here will be better able to protect their children from harm. And children reared by safety-minded parents will themselves grow up even more alert and informed about safety than their parents were.

For more information on child safety write:

National Safety Council
Child Safety Program
444 North Michigan Avenue
Chicago, Illinois 60611

Introduction

By Kenneth Jay Solomon, M.D.

Over the past few decades medicine has made remarkable progress in such difficult areas as cancer and leukemia survival and the prevention and treatment of infectious diseases. We have reached something like a 20 percent improvement in the overall mortality rate. Yet accidents still account for the greatest proportion of childhood deaths. There is even some indication that the death toll is increasing for certain groups of youngsters, most notably those between five and 14. What is responsible for these sad facts, and what can we do to give our children more adequate protection?

As a parent and pediatrician, I feel the main problem is that adults are so poorly prepared for the steps that must be taken in an emergency. I have been faced countless times with distraught, bewildered parents whose best intentions failed to aid their children because they didn't know what to do. The basic information was not readily available to them in a truly usable form.

Prevention remains our best defense against childhood accidents, but we must also know how to respond quickly and appropriately to any emergency situation as it arises. Nothing is more tragic than an emergency made worse by a parent's impulsive but misguided efforts to help the child. Hippocrates articulated the principle when he said, "First, do no harm."

This book has been carefully designed and organized for use by parents, babysitters and other laymen responsible for children's well-being. The unique indexing system on the back cover provides immediate access to guidance on how to handle just about any medical emergency your youngster may encounter. Each first-aid procedure is presented in easy to follow instructions printed in large type and is supported by clarifying step by step illustrations.

I suggest you read through the entire emergency section as soon as possible so you will have some familiarity with the recommended procedures before you ever need to use them. Remember that the basic purpose of first aid is to preserve the child's life and prevent further physical and psychological injury until help arrives. It is never a substitute for professional medical care. Since prevention is always preferable to cure, I also suggest you carefully study the opening section on preventions for the helpful guidance it has to offer. Keep the book in an accessible place known to everyone in your family.

To my knowledge, up to the present moment there has never been a handbook for parents that treated both the prevention and management of childhood emergencies. I am delighted that such a book now exists.

PART ONE

Preventions

Reducing the Odds

Parents, Children & Accidents

Accidents are by far the most common type of childhood emergency, the biggest single threat in the first 15 years of a youngster's life. Children are more likely to have serious accidents than adults because they are not only the victims but often the unconscious perpetrators. It is ironic that the major contributing factors are also some of the most basic, desirable and enjoyable characteristics of childhood itself.

During infancy the child's environment is severely limited, and it is relatively easy for parents to control its potential dangers. But as every parent learns, this phase soon ends as the baby begins to crawl and then to walk. This new mobility expands the child's world and exposes him to a greatly increased risk of injury. Yet it is normal for children to explore their new environment, to want to understand and master it with their newly developed abilities and almost limitless energy. What often places them in situations of high risk is, of course, their inexperience.

At the beginning, when your child is young and completely vulnerable, you can protect him from harm by staying physically close. But the developmental process begun at birth is designed to produce a self-sufficient, independent individual at maturity, and the child's environment must necessarily soon expand beyond the point where you can (or should) be physically present every moment of the day.

Fortunately, at about the same time the youngster's world expands, he begins to understand and respond to language. It is usually at this point that the admonition "No!" begins to be used around the home with increasing, sometimes maddening, regularity. The child's ability to respond to simple instructions is what makes it possible for you to protect him from a distance. It also enables you to begin his safety training.

Safety training involves three major steps:
● **Defining** the limits of safe behavior for the large number of threatening situations the child may be expected to encounter.
● **Teaching** these limits patiently until he understands and accepts them.
● **Reinforcing** these limits whenever he forgets or ignores them.

Consistency is an important factor in this process. It is easier for a child to follow a simple unchanging rule than one which may be altered by parental mood or whim. Restrictions that come and go according to special circumstance present younger children with confusing distinctions and subtleties that may be beyond their scope. The more clear and simple the rule, the more likely the child to abide by it.

Restrictions appropriate at one point in a child's life may become unrealistic and unnecessary only a few months later. A parent must try to strike the fine balance between the youngster's need for reasonable protection from danger and the comparable need for diversity of experience and the freedom to explore.

This is one of the most difficult responsibilities of parenthood, because the balance shifts constantly as the child's abilities and judgment improve. As the years pass, the need for parental guidance slowly decreases until, finally, the child is autonomous. As this scenario unfolds, you must be able to loosen the limitations imposed upon your child, relaxing them gradually as he demonstrates ever increasing maturity.

Yet accidents will still sometimes happen because of the child's natural tendency to test all limits. Boys and girls are aware of their ongoing physical development and constantly try to master new physical skills. Moreover, parents usually prize their child's achievements, and the youngster is encouraged by this approval to stretch out for ever new accomplishments.

The child's healthy development also requires a secure and loving environment in which he occupies an important place. To be truly effective, safety training and the discipline that comes with it should always be offered in the spirit of concern, acceptance and love. We must strive to show our children that while we may not approve of certain things **they do,** we do not disapprove of **them.**

In some households, one or both parents is particularly, even morbidly, fearful for the child's safety and tends to become overly protective. Not infrequently, a parent will have difficulty acknowledging a youngster's improved abilities, to the extent of inhibiting his normal pursuit of experience. The children of neurotically fearful parents are often insecure and profoundly lacking in confidence. Of course we should protect our children from **unreasonably** dangerous situations which have considerable potential for serious injury. Yet it is through systematic exposure to new and demanding experiences that we provide the stimulation and environmental richness essential to their ongoing development. We should want to encourage our sons and daughters to operate somewhere near the limits of their capacities without either exposing them to unreasonable danger or smothering them with our own unreasonable fears.

Home Safety

Every parent wants to give his child a safe home, a place to live and grow free of foreseeable danger. Your efforts here have a double benefit: they protect your youngster from physical harm and also establish a consciousness about safety he will take out into the world with him wherever he goes.

This chapter discusses the most prevalent kinds of home accidents and the ways they can be prevented. (Drowning, certainly one of the major hazards, is treated on pages 54-61 of the chapter on **Water Safety**.) You'll also find here room-by-room suggestions about the special dangers inherent in each different area of your home.

Remember that hazards change according to a child's age and development. Safety training is a continuing process with different requirements for each stage of childhood. Parents must not only recognize present dangers around the home but anticipate the ones to come.

Remember also that the moods and circumstances of your family have an important influence on your child's safety. Accidents are most likely to occur:

● When children are so hungry or thirsty they are ready to eat or drink anything. Many poisonings take place just before mealtime.

● When children and mothers are tired, usually before it's time for a nap, in late afternoon or before bedtime.

● When children are overactive or rushed and don't allow enough time to do things carefully.

● When mothers are pregnant or ill and not able to supervise their children with their usual patience and care.

● When parents quarrel or are under emotional stress and aren't paying adequate attention to the child. The child may react in rebellious or hazardous ways.

● When the family routine is upset by moves, long trips or vacations.

● When babysitters or other less experienced people are supervising the child.

SUFFOCATION

Because of their inexperience and relative helplessness, infants are particularly susceptible to accidental suffocation. Parents of younger children must stay constantly on the alert to this danger and learn to take the following precautions:

● Keep plastic bags out of your child's reach. Never use them as waterproof sheets or toys. They should be knotted and thrown away immediately.

● Don't give a younger child soft pillows and other bedclothes which might interfere with his breathing. Tuck the bottom sheet smoothly under the mattress and keep the top sheet loose enough to let him move about freely.

● Never leave your infant unattended with a feeding bottle propped up in his mouth.

● If you have a refrigerator or freezer stored away in your basement or garage, remove the door so your child can't be trapped inside.

● Keep storage areas uncluttered and never pile things so high they could cave in on the child.

● Put ropes, cords and long scarves where young children can't get to them.

● To prevent choking, don't let your youngster run with food in his mouth or engage in horseplay at mealtime. Make sure he doesn't put small toys and other objects in his mouth.

FALLS

Falling accidents are a major cause of serious injury around the home to children of every age. Here's what you can do to keep them to a minimum:

● Make sure your floors aren't slippery. Don't wax them to too high a finish. Wipe up spilled liquids immediately.

● Check that all carpets and scatter rugs are anchored firmly in place.

● Install non-skid rubber mats or abrasive treads inside bathtubs and showers. Use non-skid bath mats to keep your child from slipping when he steps out.

● Don't leave toys and other objects lying around the floors. Toys should be put away promptly after each use so they won't be tripped over and broken.

● Whenever you put your baby in his crib, be sure to raise the sides to their fullest height and lock them in position.

● All rooms and hallways should be lit adequately.

● Doorways and halls should be free of obstructions.

● Never leave your infant alone in a baby carrier you've placed on a table, counter, couch or chair. Stay within arm's reach and be sure to fasten his safety belt to keep him from slipping out.

● Make sure stairways remain uncluttered and in good repair. Major hazards include loose or missing handrails, loose carpeting, worn treads, poor lighting, stairs of unequal height and unanchored scatter rugs at the top of the landing. For younger children, install safety gates at the top and bottom of the stairways. Don't let your youngster run, sit or play on the stairs and keep them free of objects that don't belong there.

● Check that all balconies and high porches are in good condition and protected with strong railings.

● Open windows from the top, not the bottom, and fit them with screens with child-proof latches. Don't let your child sit on window sills or lean against the screens.

● Make sure your child's skirts and pants aren't too long and that shoes aren't too large or left untied. Never let a youngster dress up in a sash, scarf or cape that trails on the floor behind him.

● Keep your child away from table tops and other high surfaces. Don't let a toddler try to climb into his highchair by himself. Make sure to fasten the safety harness. Bunk beds are only safe for older children.

● Discourage roughhousing, bravado and wild play inside the home.

POISONING

Most poisoning accidents take place in the home and involve children under five eating or drinking toxic substances carelessly left within their reach. Almost every room in the house contains common substances that can poison a child if he ingests them:

LAUNDRY AREA
● Soaps
● Dyes
● Water softener
● Detergents
● Bleaches
● Spot remover & other cleaning solvents

GARAGE & STORAGE SHED
● Insecticides
● Solvents
● Paint thinner
● Gasoline
● Charcoal starter
● Fertilizers
● Seeds, bulbs & plants
● Pesticides
● Paints
● Paint remover
● Kerosene
● Waxes & polishes
● Weed killer

PR12

BATHROOM
- Aspirin
- Laxatives
- Rubbing alcohol
- Boric acid
- Toilet bowl cleaner
- Scouring powder
- Prescription drugs
- Witch hazel
- Epsom salts
- Drain opener
- Shampoo
- After shave lotion
- Other cosmetics & toiletries
- Ointments

BEDROOM
- Sleeping pills
- Birth control pills
- Matches & lighter fluid
- Nail polish & polish remover
- Other cosmetics & toiletries
- Aspirin & other medicines
- Contraceptive creams
- Hair spray

KITCHEN
- Drain, metal & oven cleaners
- Food extracts & spices
- Aspirin & other medicines
- Ammonia
- Room deodorizer
- Mothballs & other insecticides
- Soaps & scouring pads
- Vitamin supplements
- Cleaners & polishes for furniture, walls & floors
- Toilet bowl cleaner

WORKSHOP & HOBBY AREA
- Solvents
- Paint remover
- Chemicals
- Paints
- Glue
- Paint thinner

All these substances should be kept stored where a child can't get to them, high beyond his reach and preferably under lock and key. To prevent any possible confusion, store them separately from food and other things your child might seek out, and never keep them in soda bottles, milk cartons, coffee cans or other familiar containers. Each substance should be labeled clearly and tightly covered or capped with a child-proof lid. And never leave handbags or brief cases lying around; they may hold some of the same dangerous substances found elsewhere in the home.

The severity of a childhood poisoning may depend on the speed with which you can obtain expert emergency information and treatment. Get the telephone number of your local Poison Control Center from the phone book and write it down in the space provided on page 64. In case of an emergency, the Center will give you immediate instructions on what to do. You might also prepare yourself by having on hand the various recommended antidotes: syrup of ipecac, Epsom salts and activated charcoal. In case you are unable to reach your Center for some reason, see **POISONING,** pages 180-187, in our emergency first aid section.

FIRE AND BURNS

Fire poses a serious threat to everyone in your home as well as your children. Here are some basic measures to minimize the risk of injury:

● Be sure the electrical wiring in your home is sound.
● Never overload the circuits. Be cautious about using extension cords and multiple sockets.
● Frequently examine electric heaters, cooking equipment and other appliances to make sure they are still in good operating condition. Replace frayed cords and broken or loose plugs.
● Oily cloths and flammable liquids should be stored away from heat in closed metal containers. Rubbish should be discarded promptly.
● Be careful when you smoke.
● Use a fire screen in front of your fireplace.
● Put fire extinguishers in your kitchen and on each floor of your house.
● Install smoke detectors in rooms and hallways.
● If you live in an apartment building, make sure everyone in your family knows the proper evacuation procedures.
● If you live in a house with more than one story, install fire ladders in the upper rooms.
● Plan escape routes in advance and practice them frequently with your household. Include a meeting place outside the home where your family can assemble and be counted.

You can also protect your child against fire and burns by giving him the supervision his age requires, teaching him to avoid foreseeable hazards and taking care not to imperil him through your own carelessness.
● Make sure he understands that fires can burn and that he is to stay away from stoves, heaters, open flames, hot liquids, matches and lit cigarettes.

● Be particularly careful when you're cooking. Use the back burners whenever possible, and always turn pot handles to the rear so your child can't brush up against them or grab them. Keep highchairs away from the stove.
● At mealtime, keep hot food and drink near the center of the table where a youngster can't get at them. Never pass hot food over his head.
● Teach your child to take extreme care when turning on a hot water faucet, particularly in the shower or bath.
● Unplug electric appliances when they're not being used. When this isn't practical, make sure the cords are well out of a young child's reach so he can't chew them or pull the appliance down.
● Block off electrical outlets not in use with special plugs made for this purpose or heavy electrical tape. Teach your youngster never to stick keys, pins or other metal objects into an outlet.
● When you disconnect an extension cord from an appliance, don't leave it plugged into the wall. Your child could burn or shock himself badly if he puts it in his mouth or touches it with wet hands.
● Don't let your child use a radio, television set or other appliance around water.
● Check that all electrical toys are listed by the Underwriters Laboratory (UL) and inspect them frequently for frayed wires and loose or broken plugs.
● Teach your child what to do in a fire emergency and review it with him frequently. As soon as he's old enough, make sure he knows how to summon aid from the fire department.

GUNS

If you have guns at home, be sure to keep them unloaded and take special care to lock them safely out of your youngster's reach. Ammunition should also be locked away but in a separate storage area. Guns should always be treated as if they were loaded and never pointed at anyone.

Home Safety Tips

CHILD'S ROOM

Remove all small objects an infant might put in his mouth.

Never use plastic bags for toys or waterproof sheets.

Don't leave a pillow in the crib with your baby.

Remove large toys and boxes from the playpen. Your youngster could use them to climb out.

Make sure all the paint in the room is non-toxic.

GARAGE, BASEMENT, LAUNDRY AREA AND WORKSHOP

Teach your children to stay away from these areas. If possible, keep them locked.

Paints, solvents, insecticides and chemicals should be sealed tightly and kept beyond a child's reach, preferably in a locked storage area. Keep them in their original containers.

Remove the doors from stored refrigerators and freezers.

Potentially dangerous tools should be kept where children can't get to them. Power tools should always be disconnected when not in use.

STAIRS

Keep them well lit.

Install safety gates at the top and bottom to bar small children.

Remove all tripping hazards.

Don't let children run, play or sit on the stairs.

BATHROOM

Never leave an infant or
young child alone in a tub.

If possible, lock medicine and toiletry cabinets.
Open shelves should be high enough so your
child can't get to them. Discard old
prescription medicines.

Keep electrical appliances away from water.

Install rubber mats or abrasive treads
inside tub or shower.
Use non-skid bath mats.

Keep the door closed so your
toddler won't wander in.

SOME GENERAL TIPS

Cover unused electrical outlets with
heavy electrical tape or special plugs.

Keep children from leaning against
window screens or playing on window
sills and other high places.

Make sure to unplug an extension cord
from the outlet when you remove it
from the appliance.

Never leave an infant or
young child at home by himself.

KITCHEN

Turn pot handles toward
the back of the stove.

Household cleaners, chemicals,
bleaches and other dangerous
substances should be stored
high up and under lock and key.

Make sure knives and other dangerous
utensils stay out of reach.

Keep electrical appliances
away from water and unplugged
when not in use.

Don't place a highchair near
the stove or around such busy areas
as doorways and refrigerators.

Infant Equipment

Not all infant equipment on the market is safely designed and constructed. Here's what to look for when you shop for a crib, carriage or the like, along with some pointers about how to use them safely:

BABY CARRIERS

- The base should be wide and sturdy. Supporting devices must fasten securely to keep the carrier from collapsing.
- Check that the carrier comes with safety belts to hold the child in place.
- Attach rough-surfaced adhesive strips to the bottom to prevent it from slipping when you set it down.

BABY WALKERS

- Make sure the walker is stable and won't tip over easily. The wheel base should be longer and wider than the frame. Small, flimsy wheels or a narrow base may cause the child to fall when he leans, reaches, runs or tries to get over thresholds and rugs. Help the child past such obstacles and remove throw rugs from his path.
- Check that coiled springs and hinges are encased in protective covers. Many older style walkers are made with X frames which can catch a child's fingers. Locking devices and fasteners should be free of sharp edges and points.
- The seat should be made of unbreakable plastic or sturdy fabric with heavy-duty stitching and large, rugged snaps.

BACK PACKS

- Select the carrier appropriate to your youngster's size and weight. Make sure it is deep enough to support his back and comes equipped with safety belts.
- Leg openings should be small enough to keep the child from slipping out but large enough not to chafe his legs.
- Check for sturdy materials, strong stitching and large, heavy-duty snaps. The metal frame near his face should be cushioned with soft padding.
- Make sure the joints fasten securely and can't accidentally close on the child. Look out for points, sharp edges and rough surfaces.

CRIBS

- Check that the slats aren't so widely spaced that your infant can slip his head or body through them. The law in the United States is they can't be more than 2-3/8 inches apart.
- Bumper pads should extend around the entire crib and tie into place with at least six ties.
- Make sure the mattress fits snugly. If you can get two fingers between the mattress and the sides of the crib, it's too small.
- Look for a substantial distance between the top of the side rail and the mattress support. When your child is eventually able to stand, lower the mattress to the bottom position and lock the side rail at maximum height. You will also have to remove bumper pads, large boxes and toys, and anything else he could use to climb out. If the side is less than 3/4 of the child's height, the crib is too small for him and should no longer be used.

HIGHCHAIRS

- The chair should have a wide base to keep it stable and come equipped with a safety belt that attaches to the frame, not to the tray. Be sure to fasten the belt whenever you put your child in the chair.
- Always make sure the tray is properly latched on both sides. Don't use it as a restraining device; that's what the safety belt is for.
- Make sure the latching mechanism and the rest of the chair are free of sharp edges and points.

PLAYPENS

- Check that the slats are narrow enough to keep your child from slipping his head or body through them. They shouldn't be more than 2-3/8 inches apart. (If you have an old playpen with wide slats, interweave sheeting between them and fasten securely.)
- The weave in mesh netting should be so small that it can't catch the buttons on the baby's clothes. Large openings also make easy toeholds for climbing and could possibly strangle him should he catch his head in them.
- Make sure the floor support is sturdy enough not to collapse when your child jumps on it.
- Hinges and latches should fasten securely so they won't catch his fingers.
- Install a foam pad on the bottom of the pen. The material is long lasting and won't mildew.

STROLLERS

- Make sure the backrest is firm and nearly vertical and that the seat is firm and flat. If there is a canopy, it should clear the child's head and allow room for growth.
- Check that there are seat belts to keep the child from falling out and a brake that locks securely. Brakes on both wheels provide extra safety.
- Avoid strollers with points, sharp edges or scissors-like folding mechanisms. Latches should be out of the child's reach and must fasten securely.
- If the stroller adjusts to a reclining position, be sure it won't tip over backwards when the baby lies down.

Toy Safety

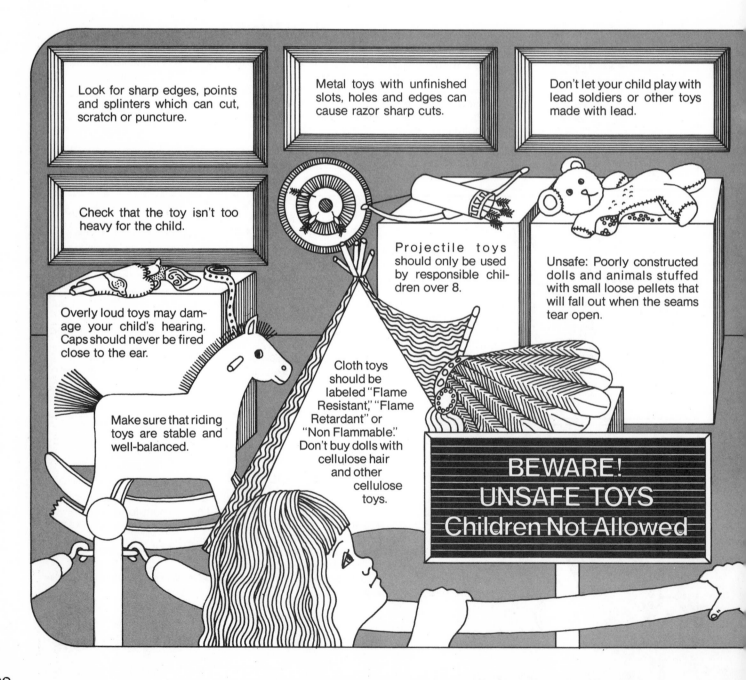

Look for sharp edges, points and splinters which can cut, scratch or puncture.

Metal toys with unfinished slots, holes and edges can cause razor sharp cuts.

Don't let your child play with lead soldiers or other toys made with lead.

Check that the toy isn't too heavy for the child.

Projectile toys should only be used by responsible children over 8.

Unsafe: Poorly constructed dolls and animals stuffed with small loose pellets that will fall out when the seams tear open.

Overly loud toys may damage your child's hearing. Caps should never be fired close to the ear.

Make sure that riding toys are stable and well-balanced.

Cloth toys should be labeled "Flame Resistant," "Flame Retardant" or "Non Flammable." Don't buy dolls with cellulose hair and other cellulose toys.

BEWARE!
UNSAFE TOYS
Children Not Allowed

All children love toys, and the playthings we give our sons and daughters benefit them a number of important ways. They teach them to focus their attention, aid their intellectual, psychological and aesthetic growth, help them develop adult skills and, of course, provide them with fun and entertainment. Unfortunately, not all these toys are safe, nor are the ways they are sometimes used.

Parents could prevent toy-related injuries more effectively if they were always caused by unsafe toys alone. There's no question that entirely too many toys **are** unsafe and account for a large portion of childhood accidents, yet other factors are usually also involved. Reputable toy manufacturers try to make their products as safe as possible, but they have to assume that parents will choose the appropriate toys for their children and give them adequate supervision. What finally determines the risk during play is a combination of the particular toy, child and circumstances and what you do (or fail to do) to protect your youngster from harm.

UNSAFE TOYS

A toy is inherently unsafe if its design or materials are defective or if there are flaws in its manufacture. Before buying a toy for your child, examine it carefully for its injury potential, looking for quality design, materials and construction throughout:

The driving springs in mechanical toys should be adequately cased. Exposed gears and mechanisms can catch fingers and clothing.

Hinged playthings should be designed to avoid crushing fingers and hands.

Don't buy electrical toys operating on house current for children under 8. Limit younger children to electrical toys that use batteries. All electrical toys should be certified safe by the Underwriters Laboratory (UL).

Toys with small parts that might be swallowed, inhaled or lodged in the ear are particularly dangerous to children under 3. The noise makers in squeak toys should be non-removable.

Cheap plastic is likely to break easily, leaving sharp or jagged edges. Flex the plastic slightly to see if it's brittle.

Toys using explosive materials are dangerous. Never let your child play with fireworks.

Toys with strings longer than 12 inches are dangerous to children under 2.

Unsafe: Dolls with clothing, hair and accessories flimsily attached with pins or staples.

LEAD BASE PAINT

Unsafe: Toys made with straight pins, easily removable nails, or wires that are or could easily become exposed.

All painted toys and paints should be labeled "Non Toxic." Make sure old toys and nursery furniture haven't been refinished with a lead base paint.

TOYS TOO OLD FOR YOUR CHILD

Toys appropriate for older children may be hazardous and frustrating for a younger child because of his inability to use them properly. Children themselves purchase 1/3 of all toys sold, so it's particularly important to teach them which playthings are—and are not—suitable for their age.

● When selecting a toy for your child, keep in mind his age, abilities, interests and limitations. Make a point of checking the manufacturer's age recommendations. Such warnings as "Not Suitable For Children Under 3 Years" are generally sound and intended to protect the younger child from toys that have small parts, break relatively easily, or for some other reason aren't safe for youngsters under the given age.

● When buying toys for older children, consider the risks to their younger brothers and sisters. Young children are always curious about the toys of their older siblings, and since they are usually unaware of the dangers, they can be seriously hurt if allowed to play with them. Teach your older children to keep their toys away from the younger kids around the house. Store toys separately for children of different ages.

BROKEN TOYS

Even reasonably well-made toys may break eventually, leaving jagged or sharp edges and points. Some apparently safe toys use hazardous prongs and knife-like points in their inner construction, which become exposed when the toy is broken.

● Select toys likely to withstand being frequently pushed, pulled at and dropped. Children like to explore how their toys are put together, and a toy should be sturdy enough to withstand their probing. Even when it breaks, it should still remain safe. Tug gently at attached parts to test their strength. Flex plastic toys slightly to see if they are brittle and likely to break easily.

● To minimize breaking (and to keep them from being tripped over), make sure that toys are put away soon after they've been played with. Indoor toys shouldn't be left outdoors, where they can be damaged by moisture and rust.

● Check your child's toys regularly to make sure they are still safe for continued use. Broken toys and children's furniture should be repaired promptly. Use only lead-free paints to restore the finish. If the toy can't be fixed, discard it.

PLAYING SAFELY

Some toy-related injuries have less to do with any defect in the toy itself than with the way it is used. Parents sometimes forget their children's inexperience and neglect the preventive measures that would keep them out of harm's way.

● Give your child the supervision and guidance his age requires:

• Children up to the age of 2 require extremely close—almost constant—supervision. By the time they are toddlers they can be taught not to walk or run with things in their mouths.

• 2 to 4 year olds are most susceptible to toy-related injuries and continue to require close supervision. This is particularly the case with boys. From this age on, they are statistically more likely than girls to have accidents. Safety training in the proper use of toys should be actively undertaken throughout these years.

• 4 to 6 year olds should be able to demonstrate more of an understanding of toy hazards and exhibit good safety practices at play. Safety training should continue.

• 6 to 8 year olds are now in school and playing further away from the direct supervision of their parents. Make sure your child has internalized the principles of safe play.

• 8 to 12 year olds may (or may not) be mature enough to play with some of the questionably safe toys they may want. Before letting your child play with chemistry sets, projectile toys, sharp tools and other potentially hazardous playthings, be certain he knows how to use them safely. Parental supervision may still be required.

● Keep an eye on your child's playmates and the way they play together. An accident may happen because a friend hasn't learned the potential dangers of a toy.

● When your youngster gets a new toy, read over the instructions with him and make sure you both understand them. Teach him the proper use of the toy, explaining the hazards which may result from its misuse. Take the time to help him develop the necessary skills.

● A toy must be given the play space it requires. Outdoor toys should only be used outdoors. Projectile toys are particularly dangerous in inadequate space.

● Check the chapter on **Bicycle Safety** for the proper use of two-wheel bikes. Your child should know the following basic safety rules for such sidewalk vehicles as coaster wagons, skate boards, roller skates, scooters and tricycles:

• Always be careful of other people, and go slowly enough to stop suddenly if you have to.

• Never fool around or show off.

• Only play on sidewalks that aren't crowded.

• Don't hold packages in your arms while you ride. Leave your arms and hands free for balancing.

• Look carefully both ways before crossing a driveway.

Toys for

UNDER 1 YEAR: Awareness of sound, motion, touch, and color. Hand to mouth curiosity. Toys should be simple, large, light in weight and brightly colored. Crib toys should be washable.

Squeak toys with noise-makers molded in
Sturdy, non-flammable rattles
Brightly colored objects hanging in view (mobiles, etc.)
Washable dolls and stuffed animals with embroidered features

Brightly colored cloth or rubber balls with textured surfaces.
Unbreakable cups and other smooth objects that can be chewed
Unbreakable teethers that can be sterilized

1 TO 2 YEARS: Age of mobility. Hand to mouth exploration. Curious.

Cloth blocks
Books with stiff pasteboard or cloth pages

Pulling toys
Nesting toys (sets of blocks, etc.)
Non-glass mirrors
Take-apart toys with large pieces

2 TO 3 YEARS: Development of language. Very curious.

Chalkboard and dustless chalk
Low rocking horse
Simple musical instruments
Simple jigsaw puzzles with large pieces
Lotto-type matching games

Wooden animals
Blocks with numbers and letters
Toys that stimulate color, size and shape identification

3 TO 4 YEARS: Vigorous physical activity. Imagination and imitation.

Manipulative toys
Sturdy trucks and non-electric trains
Toy telephone
Metal tea set
Dolls with simple wrap-around clothing
Large wooden stringing beads
Construction sets with easily connecting large pieces
Jigsaw puzzles with large pieces

Simple musical instruments
Counting frame with large beads
Peg board
Large crayons
Rugged key-wound or friction-operated toys
Blunt scissors
Lacing cards
Simple card and board games

your kids

4 TO 6 YEARS: Cooperative social play. Physical coordination.

Blocks of various geometric shapes
Picture books
Pail and shovel
Hand and finger puppets
Watercolor paints
Modeling clay
Simple kaleidoscope
Key-wound or friction-operated toys
Cut-out paper dolls

Magnetic numbers and letters
Felt board
More advanced construction toys
Kites
Stencils
Activity books
More demanding board and card games
Simple musical instruments

6 TO 8 YEARS: Independent play. Physical and intellectual interests.

Kites
Boats and planes not driven by
gasoline engines
Puppets and puppet theater
More complicated jigsaw puzzles
Games requiring some reading
Well constructed, lightweight tool sets
Dolls and doll equipment

Equipment for playing store, bank,
filling station, etc.
Magnets, magnifiers and
sets demonstrating
simple principles
of science
Flower press
Simple musical
instruments

8 TO 12 YEARS: Arts, crafts, building and science interests.

Construction models of boats, planes
and cars
Hobby material for coin and stamp
collecting, etc.
Arts and crafts kits and materials

Electric trains and other electrical toys
certified safe by the Underwriters
Laboratory (UL)
Chemistry and other science sets
Bikes and sidewalk vehicles

School Safety

By the time your child goes off to school, he is feeling a new independence and is no longer as subject to your direct supervision. The school will take on some of the responsibility for overseeing his safety, but it is crucial that you reinforce the safety lessons he learns there and show him how to protect himself from potential dangers between school and home.

GETTING TO AND FROM SCHOOL

If your child walks all or part of the way to school, map out the safest possible route, the one that exposes him to the least traffic, fewest intersections and avoids such hazards as construction sites. Emphasize that he is to follow this route and this route only, explaining why it is the safest and pointing out the hazards that do exist along the way. Make sure he understands never to hitchhike or accept rides from strangers. He should also understand the following rules of pedestrian safety. They are probably his single best protection against accidental injury.

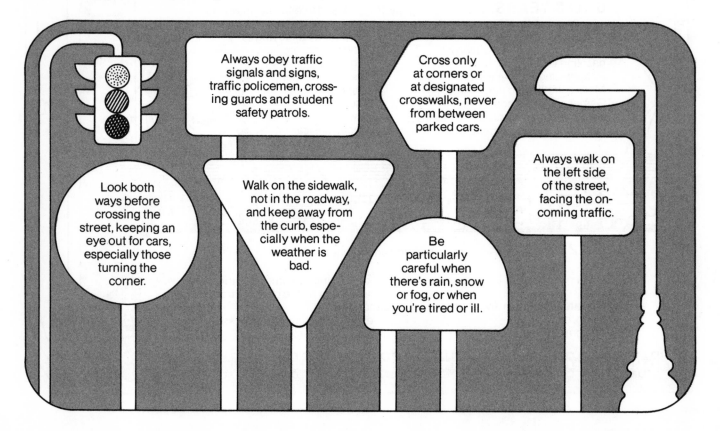

Always obey traffic signals and signs, traffic policemen, crossing guards and student safety patrols.

Cross only at corners or at designated crosswalks, never from between parked cars.

Always walk on the left side of the street, facing the oncoming traffic.

Look both ways before crossing the street, keeping an eye out for cars, especially those turning the corner.

Walk on the sidewalk, not in the roadway, and keep away from the curb, especially when the weather is bad.

Be particularly careful when there's rain, snow or fog, or when you're tired or ill.

If your youngster uses the school bus, make sure he allows himself enough time to get to the bus stop without rushing. While waiting for the bus, he should stay away from the edge of the road. If he has to cross the road to enter the bus, tell him to wait until the driver or crossing guard signals that the way is clear.

Here are some other precautions he should follow once he's gotten on board:

● Take your seat promptly and stay there until you reach your destination.

● Always obey the driver, student monitor or school safety patrolman.

● Never distract the driver or engage in horseplay.

● Don't stick your head or hands out the window or throw anything into the street.

● Make sure you know how to use the emergency exit.

If your child uses public transportation, go along with him the first few times to make certain he knows the way. He should always carry enough money to call home in case he gets lost, as well as some form of personal identification.

If you drive him to school yourself, make a point of dropping him off directly in front of the entrance so he doesn't have to cross the street. Stopping on the other side of the street needlessly exposes him to traffic and may encourage him to cross in the middle of the block.

IN SCHOOL

The classroom is probably the safest place in school because of the teacher's presence, but much of the school day is spent moving from classroom to classroom to gymnasium to cafeteria. Every school sets up safety rules to insure the safe movement of large numbers of children, and you should encourage your child to learn and obey them. It's likely that many of these precautions will be the same ones you use at home, so your youngster will already be familiar with them. But make sure he is also aware of the following basics that apply specifically to the school situation:

● Walk, do not run, in the school corridors.

● Never engage in horseplay.

● When using busy stairways, keep to the right and hold on to the hand railings. Take one step at a time. Never jump down the stairs or slide down the railings.

Tell your child to pay particular attention to the teacher's directions in woodwork and metal shop, science and photography labs, and the art and home economics rooms. Hand and power tools, kilns, stoves, chemicals and other specialized equipment can be extremely dangerous if not used in accordance with these established safety procedures:

● Always wear safety glasses when using such equipment as power saws, grinders and lathes.

● Remove rings, wrist watches, bracelets and cumbersome buckles when working around machinery. Make sure to keep neckties, scarves, loose clothing and long hair away from moving parts.

● Never remove or tamper with the safety features of a machine.

● No running or horseplay. They are particularly dangerous here.

● Keep work areas and aisles free of tripping hazards.

● Know the location and use of cutoff switches, fire extinguishers, fire blankets and other emergency devices.

Schools are particularly concerned about fire prevention. Make sure your child has a good understanding of the following safety measures:

● Never bring matches to school.

● Only use stoves, Bunsen burners and the like under a teacher's supervision.

● Always follow the teacher's directions during fire drills.

● Know how to respond quickly and correctly to the fire alarm.

● Report fires immediately to a teacher or other adult.

● Know how to use fire alarm boxes and how to telephone the fire department.

Car Safety

Automobile accidents pose the single most serious threat to your child's safety. The following preventive measures will offer a great deal of protection:

● Make sure your car stays in good operating condition.

● Take all the necessary precautions when you drive. Obey the rules of the road and stay alert for any unexpected emergencies.

● Always keep the doors locked (when you're parked as well as when you're in motion). Install child-proof safety locks on the rear doors.

● Teach your child to enter and leave the car on the passenger side only and to be careful not to catch his fingers when the door is closing.

● Don't allow him to stand on the seat or climb around when the car is in motion.

● Make sure he doesn't stick his head, hands or anything else outside the window.

● Don't allow yelling, horseplay or other distractions when you drive. If your child needs attention, pull safely off the road, then tend to him.

● Never allow him to play with the car controls, even when you're parked.

● Be sure to have on hand a first-aid kit, a flashlight with fresh batteries and emergency flares.

● On long trips, provide quiet games to keep your youngster occupied and stop at least every two hours so he can stretch his legs. Try not to travel too far in one day.

● Never leave children alone in a car for even a few minutes.

● Have the right kind of safety restraint for your child and always remember to use it.

This last point about safety restraints requires some further discussion because their importance is often overlooked. More than half the children seriously injured or killed in car accidents were not wearing safety harnesses or belts or protected by safety seats. It's simply not enough to hold your child in your arms while the car is in motion. Any sudden stop will tear him away from you and subject him to the full force of a collision.

Nor do all the safety devices on the market protect him adequately. Perhaps the worst offenders are children's car seats which merely hook loosely over the back of the regular seat. When purchasing a safety restraint for your child, check that it meets or exceeds current government standards and make certain it's the appropriate model for your child's size and age.

No safety device can offer protection if it isn't used, so be sure to place your child in the restraint for even the shortest trips. Teach him to request this protection when he's driving with someone else. If an adult safety belt is the only thing available, a small pillow should be placed between the belt and the child to serve as padding.

FROM NEWBORN TO ABOUT 20 POUNDS

Use a well padded, firmly constructed infant seat that secures to the car structure with a seat belt. The seat should be designed to stay parallel to the regular seat and preferably face backwards. Car beds are unsafe.

FROM 20 TO ABOUT 50 POUNDS

A well padded safety seat will provide protection from head-on, side and rear collisions. Make certain it is designed to be secured in place with an adult lap belt. Check that all the areas your child's head may touch are lined with padding and that there are no sharp or pointed edges anywhere on the seat. Reject models made with toy steering wheels. To protect the upper part of the body, the seat should incorporate an impact shield or restraining belts at least 1-1/2 inches wide. Also look for features that protect against whiplash injury.

OLDER AND LARGER CHILDREN

When your child outgrows the safety seat, install a lap belt that buckles firmly against his hips (not over his abdomen). If necessary, place a hard cushion under him to keep the belt low enough and allow him to see out the window. If the child is more than 4-1/2 feet tall, also use a shoulder harness. A 3-point lap and shoulder belt offers maximum protection.

Bicycle Safety

Bicycles are a wonderful source of exercise and fun, but they are not without their dangers. Too many children are injured and killed from falls and collisions that could have been avoided through proper preventive care. This chapter discusses the most common causes of childhood bike injuries and shows you how to work with your youngster to keep him safe from harm.

THE RIGHT SIZE BIKE

Bicycles are expensive, and parents sometimes buy them too large so their children can use them longer. Yet overly large bikes are one of the major causes of bicycle-related injuries. About one out of three youngsters involved in bicycle accidents was driving a bike with blocks on the pedals. When choosing a bicycle for your son or daughter, keep in mind these general guidelines about bike size and age:

AGE	5 to 7	7 to 10	Over 10
SIZE	20" wheels. Training wheels are recommended. Restrict use to sidewalks and bike paths.	24" wheels	26" wheels. Select frame size according to height and personal preference.

Bikes for beginners and young drivers should be equipped with coaster brakes rather than hand brakes, which require better coordination. Don't buy a beginner a high-rise bike; they are hard to balance.

These guidelines are rather broad, and you should go on to take a more detailed look at how the bike fits the child. To make absolutely sure it's the right size, take your youngster along to the store with you. When the two of you have narrowed down your selection, have him sit on the bike with his hands on the handlebar grips and the heel of one foot on the lower pedal, then use this illustration to check the fit:

Upper part of body is inclined slightly forward.

Hands fall naturally to the grips without stretching*

The seat is parallel to the ground or tilted only slightly upward.

Handlebar grips are at right angles to the handlebar stem and about the same height as the seat.

Thigh, calf and heel form a straight line and the knee is slightly bent.*

*after adjustments

OPERATING CONDITION AND EQUIPMENT

Many of the bicycles involved in accidents have some mechanical defect or aren't properly equipped, and these include new bikes as well as old. Make sure your child's bike has all the equipment it needs to be used safely, and periodically check it out to see whether it's still in good operating condition. Here's what to look for:

SEAT—Must be tight enough to keep its position when struck on the nose with your fist. May be raised for comfort, but after every adjustment, seat clamp bolt should be tightened until it can no longer be twisted.

HANDLEBARS—Should be tight and properly aligned with the front wheel. To check, straddle front wheel, hold wheel securely, and applying moderate pressure, try to twist handlebar and stem. Properly tightened bars should not move. Grips should always fit tightly.

REFLECTORS—For added night safety protection. Make sure they're clean. Red reflectors must be visible at night from 200 feet. White reflectors on spokes or pedals and reflectorized tape add additional safety protection. Reflectorized tires are also available.

SEAT POST—2" must remain in frame.

BELL OR HORN—Must be heard up to 100 feet. If horn is battery operated, make sure batteries work.

FRONT HEADLIGHT—Must be visible at night from 500 feet.

BRAKES—Must stop the bike quickly and smoothly.

HANDLEBAR STEM— At least 2" must remain in fork stem. (Usually the stem is stamped with a line showing maximum it can be safely raised.)

TIRES—Should be inflated to recommended pressure, usually stamped on side of tire. Valve stems should be straight. Replace worn or damaged tires.

NUTS & BOLTS—Check to be sure they're all tight.

CHAIN GUARD—Protects pants from getting tangled in the chain. Have dealer install one if bike comes without it.

PEDALS—Should turn freely and be firmly secured in the crank arms. Must be complete and undamaged. Don't use if only pedal shaft remains.

WHEELS—Should spin without significant wobble (1/16" or less). Replace any missing spokes. (Both are delicate repairs and ought to be made by a dealer.) Wheel rims should be free of dents which could interfere with proper seating of tire. For bikes with caliper brakes, sides of rims should be clean and free of oil or grease.

CHAIN—Replace or clean if noisy or rusty. When chain is in highest position, it should have only 1/2" play. If more, have dealer adjust.

BICYCLE SKILLS

It may not take your son or daughter more than a few hours to learn how to remain upright, steer and stop, but there is more to driving a bike than hopping on and pedaling away. And the cyclist is a **driver,** not just a rider. "Rider" suggests the passive role of someone only "along for the ride" and perpetuates the attitude that the bicycle is a toy. It isn't.

Most injuries to beginners come from falls. As your youngster gains experience and confidence, he'll fall a lot less, but boys and girls who have been driving for less than 2 years—typically, children about 6 to 8—are subject to a great many falling accidents. These can be minimized by enrolling your child in one of the bicycle training programs designed to teach basic driving skills. In many communities these courses are offered by the police, the "Y" and other such organizations as part of

their youth activities programs.

If such a course isn't available in your neighborhood, you can conduct your own. It will take a certain amount of effort but will give your child valuable protection and provide an enjoyable afternoon or two in the process. Youngsters are always eager to demonstrate their mastery of new skills, so it shouldn't be hard to get yours involved. And by all means have some fun with it. Make it a game to be enjoyed rather than an ordeal to be endured.

Here are nine exercises or games that will check out the basic bicycle skills your child needs to master. Space has been provided to mark off each skill as it is demonstrated. Keep in mind that these games indicate the child's control of the bike but do not prepare him to drive in traffic. We'll get to that afterwards.

NEEDED: A SCHOOLYARD, PARKING LOT OR OTHER LARGE OPEN PAVED AREA. CHALK & A PENCIL. ONE CHILD. ONE ADULT. A SUNNY DAY OR TWO. A LITTLE PATIENCE.

SCORING: 30 POINTS OR BETTER IS A GOOD PERFORMANCE.

1 BALANCE

60' (18m.)
3' (1m.)

THE CHILD DRIVES VERY SLOWLY THROUGH THE LANE:

- ☐ Taking more than 30 seconds
- ☐ Without touching the lines
- ☐ Without touching either foot to the ground
- ☐ Without using the brakes excessively

2 PEDALING & BRAKING

100' (30m.)
25' (8m.)
DISMOUNT

THE CHILD DRIVES THROUGH THE LANE AT AVERAGE SPEED:

- ☐ Keeping the balls of his feet on the pedals
- ☐ Keeping his feet parallel to the ground

AS HE APPROACHES THE END OF THE LANE, HE BRAKES THE BIKE TO A STOP:

- ☐ Without skidding
- ☐ Exerting back pressure on the rear wheel
- ☐ Keeping the pedal cranks about parallel to the ground
- ☐ Stopping about 10' from where he first applied the brake

☐ HE THEN DISMOUNTS ON THE RIGHT SIDE OF THE BIKE.

3 STRAIGHT LINE

100' (30m.)
4" (10cm.)

THE CHILD DRIVES THROUGH THE LANE:

☐ Without undue exertion
☐ Without touching the lines
☐ Without touching either foot to the ground
☐ Without skidding when he stops

4 SINGLE OBSTACLE COURSE

2' x 2' (60cm. x 60cm.)   5' (1.5m.)

FROM A MOVING START, THE CHILD DRIVES THROUGH THE COURSE, WEAVING IN & OUT AMONG THE SQUARES:

☐ Without touching either foot to the ground
☐ Without skidding
☐ Without using the brakes excessively
☐ Without undue exertion

5 DOUBLE OBSTACLE ZIGZAG COURSE

2' x 2' (60cm. x 60 cm.)   5" (13cm.)
10' (3m.)

FROM A MOVING START, THE CHILD DRIVES THROUGH THE COURSE, ZIGZAGGING BETWEEN THE SQUARES, THEN RETURNS THROUGH THE COURSE FROM THE OPPOSITE DIRECTION:

☐ Without touching the lines
☐ Without touching either foot to the ground
☐ Without skidding the rear wheel
☐ Without using the brakes excessively

6 FIGURE 8 BALANCE & STEERING

2' (60cm.)   20' (6m.)

FROM A MOVING START, THE CHILD STEERS THROUGH THE COURSE SLOWLY:

☐ Taking more than 45 seconds
☐ Making smooth & easy turns
☐ Keeping both hands on the handlebars
☐ Without undue exertion
☐ Without touching either foot to the ground
☐ Without touching the lines
☐ Without using the brakes excessively

7 TURNING AROUND

75' (23m.)
12' (4m.)

THE CHILD DRIVES DOWN 1 SIDE OF THE LANE, TURNS AROUND, DRIVES BACK & TURNS AROUND AGAIN:

☐ Without touching the lines
☐ Making smooth & easy turns
☐ Without touching either foot to the ground
☐ Without excessive braking

8 EMERGENCY STOP & TURN

20' (6m.)
6' (2m.)
3' (1m.)
2' (60cm.)

THE CHILD DRIVES DOWN THE LANE, MAKES A RIGHT TURN & STOPS, THEN DRIVES DOWN THE LANE AGAIN, MAKES A LEFT TURN & STOPS:

☐ Without touching any lines
☐ Without skidding
☐ Without touching either foot to the ground until the bike has stopped

DRIVING IN TRAFFIC

For the older child, a bicycle is not just a plaything but an important means of transportation used to visit friends, go to school, run errands, etc. As he moves from the relative safety of sidewalk and driveway out into the traffic of the street, there is a dramatically increased risk of injury from collisions with fixed objects, other bicycles, and automobiles and trucks. Since a bicycle offers no protection at all, the cyclist is the most exposed and vulnerable element in the traffic flow, and even a minor collision can have serious results.

Make certain your youngster develops a sensible attitude about using his bike in traffic and has a good understanding of traffic rules and regulations. A bicycle is considered a vehicle by law and is subject to all the traffic regulations that apply to cars and other motor vehicles. Every cyclist is expected to know these laws as well as the special regulations for bikes. You can obtain a copy of these rules at the Registry of Motor Vehicles in your community. The importance of sticking to them may be judged by the fact that 80 percent of the bicyclists killed or injured in traffic accidents were violating traffic laws at the time.

It's particularly important your child take the following precautions whenever he drives in traffic:

Safety Rules of the Road

- Drive defensively and avoid heavily traveled routes whenever possible.
- Always keep to the right and drive with the traffic, not against it.
- Use arm signals to indicate stops and turns. Indicate turns a good half block ahead.
- If it's necessary to turn left at a busy intersection, walk the bike fully across the street, then to the left after the light changes, then remount and enter traffic again from the right.
- Drive single file, keeping a safe distance from the vehicle ahead.
- Never hitch a ride from another vehicle.
- Carry packages in a basket or carrier, keeping both hands free to control the bike. Don't carry passengers, except on adult bikes fitted with special passenger seats.
- Be on the alert for car doors opening and for parked cars pulling out into traffic.
- Never stunt-ride, show off or engage in horseplay.
- Avoid driving in snow or on ice. Watch out for sand, stones, gravel, pot holes and other surface hazards.
- Don't drive fast downhill.
- Never turn or apply brakes on unstable or slippery surfaces. Coast through them in a straight line.
- In heavy traffic, dismount and walk bike across intersections, using the pedestrian crosswalk.
- For night driving use special precautions: light or white clothing, front bike light, reflectors and reflective tape.
- Wear a clip guard on trouser cuffs.

Closely check your youngster's awareness of traffic safety before allowing him to venture out into the street or travel long distances in traffic. Here is another game to help you determine his preparedness:

LEFT TURN

RETURN TO START

RIGHT TURN

DISMOUNT

REMOUNT

FINISH   **START**

DRAW A LANE 25' WIDE & 100' LONG & JOIN IT WITH ANOTHER LANE THE SAME SIZE.

CHECK HERE:

WHEN HE MAKES A RIGHT TURN DOES HE:

○ Glance back & to the left to make sure the way is clear?

○ Indicate his intention to turn by the appropriate arm signal?

○ Dismount to the right side?

○ Mount on the left side?

WHEN MOUNTING THE BIKE DOES HE:

○ Place his left foot on the pedal, which ought to be at the high point?

○ And then push off with the right foot?

○ Look first to the left?

○ And then to the right?

WHEN HE MAKES A LEFT TURN DOES HE:

○ Glance back & to the right to make sure the way is clear?

○ Indicate his intention to turn by the appropriate arm signal?

⭐ CHECK HERE UPON COMPLETION OF A PERFECT SCORE.

When you are satisfied with your child's driving skill and his knowledge of traffic regulations, it's time to test how well he performs in normal traffic.

Pick out a route about 20 blocks long that requires your youngster to turn, stop, cross intersections and, if possible, ride up and down a hill. Follow him at a safe distance in your car or, preferably, your own bike. Look for how well he demonstrates his understanding of traffic safety and how well he performs under actual driving conditions. At the completion of the drive, talk over his performance with him, calling his attention to any errors you noted.

Playground & Sports Safety

Particularly in the city, playgrounds are among the few spaces set aside for the vigorous play of childhood. Although not without their hazards, they are far less dangerous than open streets, abandoned buildings and other improvised play areas. Most playground accidents are of the minor cut, scrape and bump variety, yet more serious injuries can also occur. Not all playgrounds have the right physical environment, nor are they always safely equipped and supervised. And even in the best of them, whenever a group of children is actively climbing, swinging and jumping, there is always the possibility that someone will get seriously hurt.

This chapter sums up the most common playground dangers and the ways they can be kept to a minimum. The recommended preventions apply equally to public playgrounds and the play equipment you may have set up in your own backyard. We end with some further recommendations about sports safety, since when the child outgrows the playground he usually moves on to the athletic field and court.

THE PHYSICAL ENVIRONMENT

Before letting your child spend time in a playground, check it out yourself to make sure the play area is safe. Here's what to look for:

● The playground should be surrounded by fences to prevent younger children from wandering in and out and to allow the area to be closed off when no supervisor is present. Fences also insure that the equipment will only be approached from the proper direction.

● The equipment should be arranged according to the age group for which it is intended. Facilities for younger children should be separated from facilities for older children. This will keep the younger child away from equipment that requires a strength and skill he doesn't yet have and will protect him from being caught up in the more vigorous, potentially dangerous, activities of older kids.

● Adequate space should be marked off for each activity to protect both the participants and the passersby. Boundaries must be clearly indicated by physical barriers or painted lines. Make sure your child understands the importance of staying outside them when he's not actively playing.

● Particularly around equipment, the surface of the playground should consist of relatively soft materials such as grass, earth, sand or tanbark. Concrete, asphalt and other hard, unyielding surfaces greatly increase the chances of serious injury. Check that the surface is given the necessary maintenance to keep it safe.

● Make sure the playground is kept clear of broken glass, bottles, metal tabs from cans and other debris, especially around slides, sandboxes and swings.

PLAYGROUND EQUIPMENT

Broken down, dilapidated structures are obviously dangerous and should never be used. However, every piece of equipment used in the playground must be examined to make sure it is in good repair and safe for your child's play.

● The equipment must be firmly anchored into the ground. In most public playgrounds, the apparatus is safely embedded in concrete. Backyard equipment anchored with pegs must be checked regularly to make sure they haven't worked their way loose. All anchoring devices should be buried well below ground where they won't be tripped over.

● Check that the equipment hasn't shifted with use. Structural components designed to be horizontal or vertical must be maintained that way. Shifts in position can impose a strain on the structure which may eventually lead to its breaking or collapsing.

● Screws and bolts holding the equipment together must not be loose or missing. Exposed screws and bolts should fit flush or be capped and any protruding parts covered with tape. Fittings must be examined frequently to make sure they remain securely in place.

● Split link chains, S-hooks and similar fittings separate easily and are extremely dangerous.

● Hanging rings should either be much smaller than a child's head or much larger, under 5 inches (12.7 cm.) or over 10 inches (25.4 cm.).

● Metal structures should be kept free from rust.

● Wooden equipment should be protected against deterioration and restored or replaced as required. Check for splinters.

For a more detailed look at individual pieces of equipment, turn the page and take a tour of our Ideal Playground.

The Ideal Playground

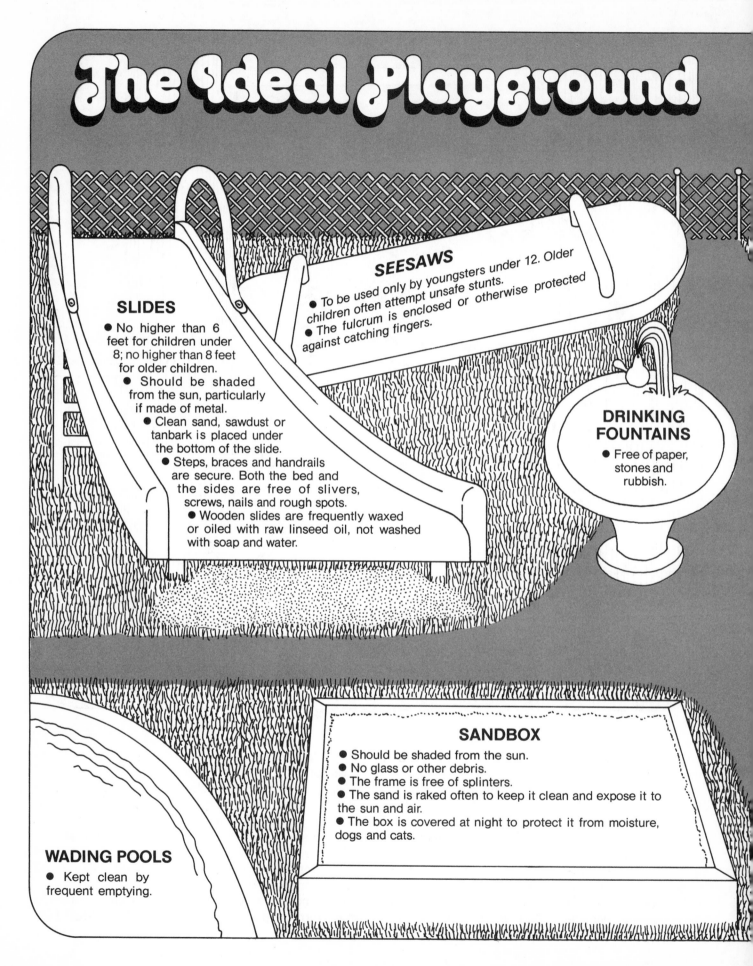

SLIDES
- No higher than 6 feet for children under 8; no higher than 8 feet for older children.
- Should be shaded from the sun, particularly if made of metal.
- Clean sand, sawdust or tanbark is placed under the bottom of the slide.
- Steps, braces and handrails are secure. Both the bed and the sides are free of slivers, screws, nails and rough spots.
- Wooden slides are frequently waxed or oiled with raw linseed oil, not washed with soap and water.

SEESAWS
- To be used only by youngsters under 12. Older children often attempt unsafe stunts.
- The fulcrum is enclosed or otherwise protected against catching fingers.

DRINKING FOUNTAINS
- Free of paper, stones and rubbish.

SANDBOX
- Should be shaded from the sun.
- No glass or other debris.
- The frame is free of splinters.
- The sand is raked often to keep it clean and expose it to the sun and air.
- The box is covered at night to protect it from moisture, dogs and cats.

WADING POOLS
- Kept clean by frequent emptying.

SWINGS

- Chair swings for kids under 5.
- Seats set at different heights for children of different sizes.
- All seats have rubber bumpers. Sling and saddle seats are the safest because they discourage youngsters from standing up.
- Worn spots and holes under the swings are filled in.

LADDERS

- Different heights for children of different ages. If the child needs help to reach it, it is too high for him.
  - Sand or other soft materials are placed underneath to cushion falls.
  - The bars do not turn when grasped.

MONKEY BARS

- To be used only by youngsters around 5 to 12 years old. Younger children should be provided with a simpler structure of interconnected bars.
- Not to be used when slippery or wet.
- The surface underneath is soft and resilient to cushion falls.
- The bars do not turn when grasped.

Playground Safety Rules

Even in our Ideal Playground, a child can be seriously injured if he doesn't use the equipment safely. Talk over these playground safety rules with your youngster and be sure he understands them.

SWINGS

- No kneeling or standing on the swings.
- Hold on tightly with both hands.
- Wait for the swing to come to a full stop before getting off. Never jump off.
- Don't hold anyone on your lap or ride double.
- Never climb the supports.

DRINKING FOUNTAIN

- Fooling around at the fountain can cause broken teeth.

WADING POOL

- Never go wading if you're overheated, sick or have a skin infection.

SEESAWS

- Hold on tightly with both hands and sit facing each other.
- Keep your hands and feet out from under the board as it nears the ground.
- Don't stand or run on the board.
- Never bump the board on the ground.
- Warn the other person before getting off.
- To get off, hold the board tightly and let it rise gradually until the other child has his feet on the ground.

SLIDES

- Climb one step at a time, keeping a safe distance from the child in front of you.
- Only one person should slide down at a time. Slide sitting up with your feet in front of you. Don't hold on to the sides.
- Quickly move away from the bottom of the slide.
- Don't try to crawl or run up the slide or slide down backwards.
- Never go sliding in a wet bathing suit.

SANDBOX

- For younger children only.
- Don't take food into the sandbox.
- No sharp or pointed playthings should be brought into the sand.

LADDERS

- Don't use a ladder if you can't reach it by yourself.
- Climb in one direction only, either up or down.
- Don't put your head or feet through the rungs.

- No Pushing.
- No Fighting.
- No Dogs.
- No Bikes.
- Never play with the equipment when it's wet or icy.

Buying Backyard Equipment

- Only buy equipment that matches your child's age, size and physical abilities.

- The more versatile the pieces, the better. Children have a short attention span.

- If the equipment doesn't come fully assembled, be sure there are clear but detailed instructions on how to set it up.

- Place the equipment at least 6 feet away from fences, walls and other obstructions.

- Install it over grass, sand, soft earth, etc., never over concrete or other hard surfaces.

- Make sure the equipment is stable. It should come with anchoring devices to hold it firmly to the ground.

- Don't buy structures with sharp edges, rough surfaces or open ended hooks.

- Check that all nuts, bolts and clamps are tight.

SPORTS

When a youngster outgrows the playground, he usually turns to sports to satisfy his need for excitement and challenging physical activity. Every sport has its own special hazards and benefits, but the principles of accident prevention are essentially the same for all of them:

- The playing area should be large enough to keep children from running into walls and other obstacles, with sufficient space around it to let other people pass by safely. Goal supports and other obstructions that can't be removed must be well padded to reduce injuries from accidental collisions. Playing surfaces should be smooth and even.

- The child should be provided with the equipment the game requires: body padding, cleated shoes and a helmet for tackle football, basketball sneakers for basketball, etc. If your youngster wears eyeglasses, make sure he has unbreakable lenses or eyeglass guards.

- The child should be in the proper physical condition and have practiced the basic skills the sport requires. When he is prepared for the demands of the game, he is less likely to suffer accidental injury and will also enjoy himself more. The greater the inherent risk of injury in a sport, the more time should be given to preparation. Remember that youngsters often attempt things beyond their strength and skill and that every athletic activity makes its own unique demands on coordination, stamina and judgment.

- Don't let your child play with a sore arm or leg, and encourage him to play different positions over the course of an afternoon, particularly if he likes to catch or pitch. Children's bones are soft and vulnerable and can be damaged by constant strain. For the same reason, never push a child beyond his capabilities or endurance.

- Competitive sports should always involve children of about the same age, size and physical skill. This will minimize the risk of injury and allow everyone to develop a sound attitude about competition by enjoying at least some success.

- The child should have a good general awareness of sports safety as well as an understanding of the hazards of a particular activity. Before allowing him out on the playing field, make sure he appreciates the importance of placing the safety of self and playmates above everything else. Ask him to identify the potential dangers in a given sport and call his attention to any he may have overlooked.

47

HIKING

Hiking is a simple, enjoyable recreation that provides excellent exercise and gets your youngster outdoors into the world of nature. The following precautions will keep his hiking experiences safe as well as pleasurable:

● The length and difficulty of the hike should always match the child's age and skill. Young or new hikers should start off with short walks along a road or clearly marked trail. Long hikes over unmarked, rough terrain are best left to older, more experienced children.

● Make sure your youngster has the necessary supervision or companionship. Solo hikes should be reserved for older children who have demonstrated their mastery of hiking skills. Until then, it's best to have at least three people along on an outing. The companionship adds to the fun, and in case of an accident, someone can stay with the injured child while a third person goes for help.

● All hikes should be planned and prepared for in advance. The longer the hike and the rougher the terrain, the more planning and preparation that are required. For even short outings, you should know where your child is going and when to expect him back. Be sure he understands never to set out on a hike without your knowledge and approval.

● See to it that your child is properly dressed to protect himself from sun and insects and unexpected changes in weather. He should always carry a water repellent jacket or poncho in case of rain.

● Footwear should be appropriate to the length of the hike and the terrain to be traveled. Rubber and other flexible soles provide good footing in the woods, but leather soles are too slippery. Boots are essential for rough ground. Sneakers and other low laced shoes are satisfactory for roads or improved trails.

● Shoes and boots should fit comfortably and already be broken in. Treat new boots with one of the various waterproofing products specifically designed to make them water repellent. To prevent blisters, check that the child's heels don't slip when he walks. Two pairs of socks are preferable. The inner layer should be orlon or cotton and the second pair thick wool.

● A peaked cap will help keep the rain and sun out of your child's eyes. Sunglasses also add comfort and protection.

● Your youngster should carry along with him all the food and drink he'll need. For a short outing, a canteen (not a glass jug) of water, a sandwich and an apple or orange should suffice. Unless he is extremely knowledgeable about woodlore, he should never eat fruit, nuts, berries or other vegetation found along the way. They might well be poisonous.

● Even on a short hike, your child should always take along a first-aid kit to deal with cuts, scrapes and blisters as well as more serious emergencies. Check that it contains such basic items as adhesive bandages and sterile dressings.

● He should also carry a compass and a map of the area and know how to use them. Emphasize that until he learns these skills, he is never to hike alone or leave the marked path or road. A flashlight is also helpful for reading road signs and avoiding bad footing when it gets dark.

● Teach your youngster not to panic or wander about aimlessly if he gets lost, but to stay where he is until help arrives. Explain to him that when he doesn't get back home when expected, a search party will look for him along the route he originally projected. He should always carry a whistle among his emergency supplies and know the universal distress signal—three short blasts repeated frequently. The signal will help rescuers find him even in darkness.

● Make sure he understands the dangers of lightning and never to seek shelter under a tall tree, especially if it stands alone in a clearing or is higher than the trees around it. If he's caught in the woods during a storm and can't find any other protection, the safest spot is under a group of young trees of about the same height. In open countryside, he should look for a protected spot away from anything tall.

● Your youngster should never approach a strange dog or other animal he might encounter in the woods or along a country road. If a dog comes up to him, he should stand still with his hands at his sides, let the dog sniff him to get his scent and speak to it in a calm, low voice. Sudden movements, yelling or running away will only increase the chance of attack.

CAMPING

After gaining some experience in hiking, many youngsters want to begin camping out in the woods for several days at a time. Camping requires greater preparation, more elaborate equipment and specialized knowledge and skills. Initial trips should be made with parents or other adults or as part of organized youth activities. Before letting your child camp out, make sure he is in good physical condition and doesn't have a cold or other ailment which might be aggravated by sleeping outdoors. If he has any special medical problems, consult his doctor to see what safeguards are required. Here are some other basic precautions that will insure his comfort and safety:

● Find out as much as you can in advance about the camping area. Talk with people who have already camped there for their suggestions and warnings. Obtain a detailed map of the area so your youngster can familiarize himself with such major features of the countryside as mountains, valleys, swamps, rivers and streams. The map will also help him choose the best routes and camp sites and steer him away from natural or man-made hazards. Superior inexpensive maps of the United States are available from the United States Geological Survey, G.S.A. Building, U.S. Department of the Interior, Washington, D.C. 20242. (Road maps are made for drivers and don't usually show the details a camper needs.)

● Work out a timetable with your child so you'll know where he'll be at various times and when he'll return home. Stress the importance of sticking to this schedule. He should also have an alternate plan in case the weather turns out unsuitable for camping.

● While your youngster shouldn't be overloaded with equipment, he should certainly take along everything he will need for his enjoyment and safety. This will vary according to the length of the outing, the character of the countryside and the weather likely to be encountered, but the basics include:

• Food and water. Depending on his size, a child requires between one and two pounds of food a day. Cans are bulky and heavy and glass jars break, so dehydrated foods are the best alternative. Have your child sample them at home first to be sure he finds them palatable.

• A change of clothes, a warm sweater, extra socks, a cap and a waterproof jacket or poncho. It's always safest to assume it will be cold and damp at night and rainy during the day.

• Sleeping and cooking equipment: a tent or tarp, a warm, lightweight sleeping bag, a ground pad and nylon ground cloth, a canteen, eating utensils, a collapsible cup, a cooking pot, aluminum foil, a good folding saw and several waterproof containers of matches to be carried in different pockets. Meals should be simple to prepare but nourishing and tasty.

• A first-aid kit, insect repellent, soap, a toothbrush and other toilet equipment, a pocket knife, whistle and a compass and map.

● A camp site should always be selected well before nightfall. Tell your child to look for a level spot out in the open, preferably near good water and firewood. It should be somewhat higher than its surroundings so water will drain away if it rains.

● See to it that he knows how to build a campfire safely. The area 10 feet around the fire should be cleared of grass, brush and anything else that might accidentally ignite, and the fire should be no larger than necessary for cooking and warmth. If he builds it in a shallow pit he has dug in the ground, the wind won't scatter the embers. Tents should be set up a safe distance from the fire and one or two buckets of water kept nearby as a safety measure.

● Check that your youngster's tent is light in weight, easily assembled and fire retardant. No tent is truly fireproof, so he should never light a campfire or camp stove inside it. Nor should he use paraffin or kerosene to make it water repellent since this will make it more flammable. Show him how to use it properly and keep it in good repair. The fine netting provided to keep out mosquitoes and other insects will work well if it is kept tightly closed and free of holes.

● A camper shouldn't attempt to feed or play with any animals he may come across. In the woods, all animals are wild, and no matter how cute or friendly they seem, they can inflict nasty bites and scratches. Large animals usually avoid humans, but raccoons, skunks, porcupines and the like may visit the camp, particularly if food or garbage is left in the open. If the camp is kept clean at all times, they'll have little reason to come around.

● Make sure your youngster can recognize poisonous snakes and knows to stay away from them. Photocopy the emergency treatment for **SNAKE BITE** on pages 94-95 and put it in his first-aid kit.

COPPERHEAD

CORAL SNAKE

RATTLESNAKE

WATER MOCCASIN

Water Safety

The principal danger from water is, of course, drowning, a tragic mishap that claims thousands of young lives each year. Many, perhaps all, these children might have been saved if their parents had been better informed and taught them how to stay out of harm's way. This chapter details the most common causes of childhood drowning accidents and the recommended preventions. After reading it yourself, we suggest you review it with your youngster, your babysitter and anyone else who shares responsibility for your sons' and daughters' safety.

Access gates should swing shut automatically and latch securely, with the latch well beyond a child's reach. Keep the gates locked when the pool isn't being used. Give your neighbors spare keys or the lock combination so they can get in quickly if you're away.

Surround the pool with fences or other barriers to keep youngsters from wandering in alone. Construct them at least 4 feet high, with the supports on the pool side so a child can't climb over easily.

Install artificial lighting for nighttime emergencies. Use wiring approved by the Underwriters Laboratory (UL). Installation should be made by a competent electrician.

AROUND THE HOME

For infants, toddlers and younger children, the best protection against drowning accidents around the home is close adult supervision. Never leave a baby alone near water for even the briefest moment. A drowning accident can take only a few seconds. If you're bathing your child and the telephone or doorbell rings, wrap him in a towel and bring him with you while you tend to it. When he becomes old enough not to need constant watching, continue to stay nearby, keeping an ear tuned to the sounds of his talk and play.

Full bathtubs and wading pools are obvious hazards, but even a scrub bucket, diaper pail or vaporizer can be dangerous. If there's enough water to cover an infant's or toddler's nose and mouth, there's enough to drown him. Your child may be attracted to the light shimmering on the surface, the sound of water running or by something floating on top. His curiosity aroused, he may tumble in headlong and not have the strength or coordination to pull himself out. To prevent this sort of accident, never draw water until you are ready to use it, never leave it within your child's reach, and discard it as soon as you're done with it. Always keep the lids on diaper pails, drain scrub buckets and store them away promptly, and empty bathtubs when they're not being used.

Outdoors, don't let your child play around cesspools, puddles and ditches. Empty small wading pools after each use and turn them over or deflate them to keep rain from collecting.

Many drowning accidents around the home take place in larger backyard swimming pools, so the following precautions are particularly important:

● Keep the pool covered during the months it isn't in use. Rigid covers are preferable to flexible models because they won't collect rain.

● Teach your child never to play in any pool away from home without your knowledge and approval. Fully 1/3 of all childhood drownings occur in the pools of neighbors.

● If there's a pond near your home, make sure the safe swimming areas are marked off and the danger points indicated with warning signs. The pond should be supplied with the same rescue devices shown below for pools:

Post the location of the nearest telephone, the numbers to call in an emergency (the local rescue or emergency squad, ambulance, doctor) and instructions for water rescue and artificial respiration. Photocopy pages 124-127 and 144-145. Hang them inside a shed or keep them in a waterproof can at poolside.

The pool should be equipped with basic rescue devices kept stored in a shed or other protected area and reserved for emergency use only. Include a floatable pole longer than 1/2 the pool's width, a ring buoy attached to a rope and a first-aid kit.

SWIMMING

The single best protection against drowning is knowing how to swim. With professional instruction, most children can begin learning at a very early age, and the younger they start the better. Good programs are offered by the Red Cross, the Boy and Girl Scouts, the "Y" and other community organizations. If your child isn't ready to swim, he can still learn to float.

Even good swimmers under the age of 12 or so still need adult supervision. Infants, toddlers and young non-swimmers require it constantly. Don't let a lifeguard do your watching for you, particularly in a crowded pool. Make sure you're not responsible for so many small children that you can't keep track of all of them all the time. Never let a toddler run loose near a pool. Pool decks are often slippery, and he could easily fall in. It's best not to let a non-swimmer enter the water without you, and you should certainly always keep him within immediate reach.

Know the water you're letting your child play in.

Check out an unfamiliar pool before letting your youngster use it. Enter the shallow end and walk toward the deep end to determine the depths, traction and slope of the bottom. Make sure pool slides and diving boards are well constructed and in good shape. Pool ladders and stairs should be equipped with hand rails on both sides. Before allowing a non-swimmer to enter the water, make certain it really is shallow enough for him to stand in comfortably, without unexpected sharp drop-offs or an irregular or slippery bottom. He should never go out over his head, and should only use inflated tubes, rafts and waterwings with adult supervision. They build false confidence and may drift him into deep water.

Your child should know the rules for playing safely in the water by the time he is old enough to go off to a pool or beach without you. Make sure he learns and understands the following precautions:

Never go swimming alone. Always use the "buddy system."

When swimming with a group, choose someone as lookout to oversee everyone's safety, even if a lifeguard is present.

Swim only in protected areas. Obey the posted rules and the lifeguard's instructions. Never swim in a public beach if there isn't a lifeguard present. Don't swim where people are actively engaged in water sports.

Before wading, swimming or diving in an unfamiliar place, find out the depth of the water and whether there are any strong currents, sudden dropoffs or hidden rocks, branches or roots. Stay out of very cold or fast moving water and watch out for undertows.

Don't engage in horseplay, roughhousing or showing off.

Check that diving boards and pool slides are sturdy and not slippery. Make sure the water underneath them isn't too shallow. Never run on diving boards or dive off the sides. Learn how to dive properly.

Always pay attention to the weather. Stay out of the water if it's going to storm.

Know your limitations and never push yourself beyond them.

Never swim when you are tired, overheated or chilled.

Wait at least an hour after eating before you enter the water.

Before swimming in the ocean, find out about the changes in the tides and whether there's any danger of sharks or poisonous marine life. Remember that ocean swimming is much more difficult and exhausting than fresh water swimming.

Be careful about hyperventilating before swimming under water. Excessive deep breathing can inactivate the body's warning signals — that you need a fresh breath, and you may black out before you can surface.

Never dive from rocks or under buoys or boats.

If you find yourself in trouble in deep water, stay calm and think out the best plan of action.

BOATING

Particularly for younger children, the boating environment is filled with hazards—poisons, gas cans, sharp objects, low doorways and ceilings, stairways, ropes, holes, protrusions, etc. Always check it out carefully and watch your child closely to keep him out of trouble.

Know where poisonous substances are kept and make sure they are securely closed and placed where your child can't get to them. Sharp objects should be stored out of a youngster's reach and ropes kept where he can't get tangled up in them. Keep him away from stairways and places where he might trip or fall or bump into protruding objects. Stairways should always be closed off when not in use.

When you take your child out on a boat, continue to supervise him carefully and be sure you're prepared for any emergency. There should be personal flotation devices (PFD) for everyone on board, and non-swimmers should wear them constantly. Your youngster's PFD should fit him snugly enough to keep him from slipping out. Make sure that for every child who doesn't swim there's an expert swimmer who will keep an eye on him. Take a first-aid kit with you as well as rescue lines or life preservers. Check that you have bailing cans and that a motor boat is equipped with a fire extinguisher.

Before a child takes out a boat himself, he should be a skilled swimmer and understand all the above precautions. It's equally important that he knows the following basics of safe boating:

- Know how to handle the boat. Learn from a qualified person. Before taking it out in deep water, put in the necessary hours practicing near shore. Know how to right a capsized canoe and climb back into it and how to handle a boat in a sudden squall or storm.

- Be sure the boat is in good repair and properly equipped.

- Know the water you are boating in.

- Never overload a boat. Distribute the weight evenly and keep it low. Keep the passengers down to a safe number.

- Never smoke around fuel. Closed in fueling areas must be ventilated before a motor boat is started, and all fuel spills wiped up promptly.

- Know how to conduct yourself safely on board. Never engage in horseplay or showing off. Be careful around slippery decks. Don't stand upright in a canoe or rowboat. A youngster should always sit toward the middle of a rowboat or motor boat, never in the bow, where any sudden movement could knock him into the water.

- Know about right-of-way rules, channel markings, anchorages, the correct use of lights and the relevant boating laws.

- Never go out if there's a chance of storm. Check the weather forecasts in advance.

- Have a plan of travel and leave this information with someone on shore.

WATER SKIING, SURFING, SNORKELING AND SCUBA DIVING

These water sports involve many of the same dangers as swimming and boating as well as their own special hazards. Before letting your child take part in them, make sure he understands these fundamentals:

- Know how to swim expertly and be in good physical condition. Don't scuba dive if you have a respiratory ailment.

- Learn the basics of the sport from a qualified teacher. Build up your skills gradually without trying to do too much at once. As with swimming, know your limitations and don't push yourself beyond them.

- Never use restricted areas. Keep away from swimmers and stay conscious of other water skiiers, surfers and divers.

- Make sure your equipment is in good shape, particularly for scuba diving.

- When water skiing, wear a PFD and have a third person along to keep watch and pass your signals to the driver.

- Don't go out in bad weather or rough water.

FISHING

Fishing is much more reposeful than surfing or water skiing, but it is not without its dangers. Your child should pay attention to the following precautions:

- Carry your fishing rod disassembled if possible. Keep hooks and plugs secured to a hook keeper on the rod or cover the barbs with cork.

- Never wade into a stream, lake or pond by yourself. There may be underwater shelves, holes or other sudden drops into deep water. Test each step in advance, keeping most of your weight on the foot that's already grounded. Be on the alert for stumps, roots and other tripping hazards.

- Maintain plenty of distance between yourself and other fishermen.

- Never fish where people are swimming.

- When baiting a hook, keep a firm grip on the bait. Hold the fish securely when you remove the hook.

- Know what to do if a fishhook becomes impaled. Photocopy pages 108-109 and carry them in your tackle box along with the necessary first-aid supplies.

SURVIVAL TECHNIQUES

Even an experienced swimmer may sometimes find himself in danger and should know how to cope with it beforehand. The following survival techniques will help your child through most emergencies. Talk them over with him and, where possible, practice them together in a pool until he has them mastered. Knowing what to do in advance will build up his confidence and decrease the chance of panic. His survival could depend on his ability to remain calm and bring himself to safety quickly.

● **Cramps:** Every swimmer occasionally experiences a cramp, a painful muscle contraction which greatly impedes the body's movement. Make sure your child understands a cramp need not be serious if he keeps calm and takes proper action. When he feels his muscle tighten, he should take a deep breath, roll to a face-down position in the water and grasp the cramped area firmly with one or both hands **(Figure 1)**. Continued firm pressure will release the cramp and permit him to move to land. He can also ease a leg cramp by straightening his leg and forcing his toes upward toward the knee **(Figure 2)**. Cramps are most likely to occur when muscles are tired and the water is particularly cold, good reasons for making swims relatively short at the start of the summer.

Figure 1   Figure 2

● **Drownproofing:** Should your child ever find himself caught out in deep water, the following technique will keep him afloat and conserve his energy between active efforts to reach safety or until help arrives:

1 Take a breath through your mouth and allow yourself to sink below the surface. Hang there loosely with your arms, legs and head relaxed. The air in your lungs will bring you effortlessly back to the surface.

2 When your head is partly out of water, stretch out your arms and at the same time move one leg forward and the other back, as in a scissors kick.

3 To take a fresh breath, gently pull your arms downward toward your hips and bring your legs together, pressing against the water with your soles and heels. As soon as your arms start downward (not before),

begin to exhale through your nose and continue exhaling until your nose rises above the surface. Be sure to keep your eyes open. Then exhale through your mouth. Your chin should be right on the water, not above it.

4 Just as your head goes under again, give a slight downward push with your arms or legs or with both of them together. This will keep you from sinking too deeply.

5 Rest underwater completely relaxed. Stay under until you would **like** a fresh breath, not until you absolutely **must have** one.

If the child becomes chilled, he can conserve his body warmth by drawing his arms and legs up to his chest and keeping his head above water.

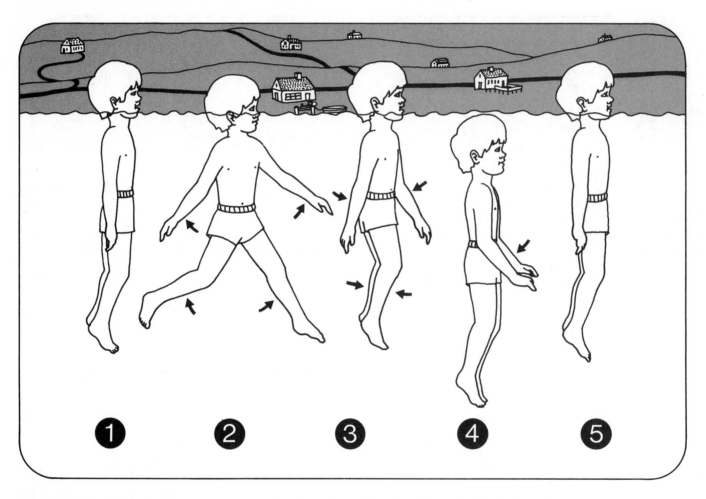

● **Improvising A Float:** Show your youngster how he can use such clothing as his trousers or shirt to help stay afloat in an emergency. Air forced into wet clothing will form a buoyant air pocket that will last as long as it is kept submerged.

To inflate a shirt or jacket, button it to the neck, hold the lower front out and away from your body with one hand, then cup your other hand and drive it down into the water, letting the air trapped in your palm escape out of the water and into the garment. Repeat the process until an air pocket forms, and replenish

the air as it gradually leaks out.

Trousers work even better because they can hold more air. To inflate a pair of pants, **1** take them off, close the zipper, and knot each leg at the cuff. **2** As you tread water, hold the pants at the waist, swing the legs behind your head, then quickly whip the waist down into the water, trapping the air in the legs. Take a relaxed floating position and use small underwater strokes. **3** Or lie on your back, holding the float to your chest while kicking with your feet.

● **Capsized Boats:** Teach your child to stay near a boat that has capsized or flooded. Even when submerged a few inches under the surface, it will probably continue to float because of its natural buoyancy or the air trapped inside. A youngster can conserve his strength until rescue arrives by clinging to the bottom of an overturned boat, and by kicking with his feet as he holds on he may be able to propel himself back to land. It is also possible to sit within a boat that has become completely flooded and paddle back to safety with your hands. Floating objects from a capsized boat —a thermos jug, oar, life preserver, etc.—can also help you back to shore. You can gain additional flotation as you hold on by keeping only your nose above water.

● **Strong Currents:** A river current can be exceedingly strong and may easily carry a young swimmer away from land. Make sure your child knows that if he is caught in a strong current he will probably exhaust himself if he tries to fight it. Instead, he should swim diagonally across the current with its flow, even though he may come to land some distance away. Most river currents make their way closer to shore eventually.

● **Broken Ice:** Should your youngster ever break through the ice while skating or playing on the frozen surface, he shouldn't try to climb out immediately. If the ice is thin or weakened, his efforts will only break more of the ice and subject him to repeated dunkings. Rather, he should kick his feet to the surface and to the rear to avoid going under the ice, extend his hands and arms in front of him onto the unbroken ice and slide forward onto the solid surface. If the ice breaks again, then continue to slide forward until the ice is firm enough to give the needed support. To distribute his weight over the widest possible area, he should remain prone as long as the ice is still thin and inch himself along in that position, rather than stand upright and put his full weight on one small area.

● **Helping Someone In Trouble:** Besides knowing how to save himself from drowning, your child should also know how to rescue someone else without jeopardizing his own safety. Unless he is fully trained in lifesaving techniques, he should never try to swim to the aid of a drowning person. Instead, he should use the following methods of assistance, which are also treated on pages 144-145:

• Near shore, use a reaching assist. Drop to the ground, extend your head and chest over the water and reach out a hand to the person in trouble. If you can't reach him without losing your own balance, reverse the position and extend your legs while holding on to a branch or other firm handhold.

• If the person is just out of body reach, look around for something else to reach him with—a stick, fishing pole, rope, etc. A shirt or coat held by the sleeve may be long enough to pull him to safety. Even if the person is underwater, as long as he is still conscious, he will instinctively grasp anything thrust into his hands or pushed against his chest.

• Find a float. Anything buoyant—a thermos, board, log, buoy, oar, boat, etc.— that can be gotten within reach of a drowning person can provide at least momentary relief while you seek further help.

Emergency Medical Information

These pages provide an immediate overview of your youngster's medical history and can save valuable time in an emergency. If you have more than two children, make as many extra photocopies as you need and tape them into the book. You should also give copies to your children's teachers, camp counselors and the other adults with whom they spend significant time. Be sure to keep the information current.

CHILD'S NAME _____ DATE OF BIRTH _____
ADDRESS _____ HOME PHONE _____
FATHER'S PHONE AT WORK _____ MOTHER'S PHONE AT WORK _____

PEDIATRICIAN: NAME _____ OFFICE PHONE _____ HOME PHONE _____
FAMILY DOCTOR: NAME _____ OFFICE PHONE _____ HOME PHONE _____
ALTERNATE DOCTOR: NAME _____ OFFICE PHONE _____ HOME PHONE _____
DENTIST: NAME _____ OFFICE PHONE _____ HOME PHONE _____
MEDICAL INSURANCE: COMPANY NAME _____
ADDRESS _____ POLICY NUMBER _____

DATES OF MOST RECENT IMMUNIZATIONS

TETANUS _____ DIPHTHERIA _____ POLIO _____
MEASLES _____ OTHER _____

BLOOD TYPE _____
RH FACTOR   RH NEGATIVE _____
(CHECK ONE)   RH POSITIVE _____

PRESENT MEDICAL PROBLEMS & CHRONIC CONDITIONS (EPILEPSY, ASTHMA, ETC.)

_____ _____ _____
_____ _____ _____

ALLERGIES (DRUGS, INSECT BITES, ETC.)

_____ _____ _____
_____ _____ _____

MEDICINES TAKEN REGULARLY

NAME _____ REASON TAKEN _____ DOSE & FREQUENCY _____
NAME _____ REASON TAKEN _____ DOSE & FREQUENCY _____
NAME _____ REASON TAKEN _____ DOSE & FREQUENCY _____

SPECIAL PRECAUTIONS & OTHER INFORMATION _____
_____
_____

	NATURE	DATE	DOCTOR	PHONE
HOSPITALIZATIONS				
SURGERY				
MAJOR INJURIES				
PSYCHIATRIC CARE OR COUNSELING				

Emergency Medical Information

CHILD'S NAME _____ DATE OF BIRTH _____
ADDRESS _____ HOME PHONE _____
FATHER'S PHONE AT WORK _____ MOTHER'S PHONE AT WORK _____

PEDIATRICIAN: NAME _____ OFFICE PHONE _____ HOME PHONE _____
FAMILY DOCTOR: NAME _____ OFFICE PHONE _____ HOME PHONE _____
ALTERNATE DOCTOR: NAME _____ OFFICE PHONE _____ HOME PHONE _____
DENTIST: NAME _____ OFFICE PHONE _____ HOME PHONE _____
MEDICAL INSURANCE: COMPANY NAME _____
ADDRESS _____ POLICY NUMBER _____

DATES OF MOST RECENT IMMUNIZATIONS

TETANUS _____ DIPHTHERIA _____ POLIO _____
MEASLES _____ OTHER _____

BLOOD TYPE _____
RH FACTOR   RH NEGATIVE _____
(CHECK ONE)   RH POSITIVE _____

PRESENT MEDICAL PROBLEMS & CHRONIC CONDITIONS (EPILEPSY, ASTHMA, ETC.)

_____ _____ _____
_____ _____ _____

ALLERGIES (DRUGS, INSECT BITES, ETC.)

_____ _____ _____
_____ _____ _____

MEDICINES TAKEN REGULARLY

NAME _____ REASON TAKEN _____ DOSE & FREQUENCY _____
NAME _____ REASON TAKEN _____ DOSE & FREQUENCY _____
NAME _____ REASON TAKEN _____ DOSE & FREQUENCY _____

SPECIAL PRECAUTIONS & OTHER INFORMATION _____
_____
_____

	NATURE	DATE	DOCTOR	PHONE
HOSPITALIZATIONS				
SURGERY				
MAJOR INJURIES				
PSYCHIATRIC CARE OR COUNSELING				

Emergency Telephone Numbers

This list of emergency numbers should be filled in immediately, then photocopied so you can also post it next to your telephone. Keep the numbers up to date.

Be sure to show it to your babysitter whenever you go out.

POLICE _____ RESCUE SQUAD OR EMERGENCY AMBULANCE

FIRE DEPARTMENT _____ _____

POISON CONTROL CENTER _____ HOSPITAL EMERGENCY _____

PEDIATRICIAN: NAME _____ OFFICE _____ HOME _____

FAMILY DOCTOR: NAME _____ OFFICE _____ HOME _____

ALTERNATE DOCTOR: NAME _____ OFFICE _____ HOME _____

DENTIST: NAME _____ OFFICE _____ HOME _____

NEAREST DRUGSTORE _____ ALL NIGHT DRUGSTORE _____

FATHER'S PHONE AT WORK _____ MOTHER'S PHONE AT WORK _____

NEIGHBORS   NAME _____ ADDRESS _____ PHONE _____
& FRIENDS:

                NAME _____ ADDRESS _____ PHONE _____

TAXI _____ EMERGENCY SHELTER _____

ELECTRIC COMPANY _____

GAS COMPANY _____

OIL COMPANY _____

WATER DEPARTMENT _____

OTHER NUMBERS _____

_____

Stocking Up: First-Aid Supplies

Every household should have a first-aid kit stocked with the basic supplies necessary for treating childhood emergencies. You can put your own kit together by purchasing the individual items listed on this page. Check off each item as you place it in the kit. If you prefer to buy a commercial kit that is already assembled, use this list to make sure its contents are complete. Always keep the kit stored in the same place, well out of a youngster's reach, and be sure your family and babysitter know where to find it. Keep it fully stocked and replace supplies as they are used.

You should also have first-aid kits for your car or boat and for hiking and camping expeditions. For hiking and camping, you might also buy a special snake bite kit containing a constricting band, sterile blades and a suction device. If your child has severe allergic reactions to insect bites and stings, have his doctor prescribe an insect sting kit and keep it with your other emergency supplies.

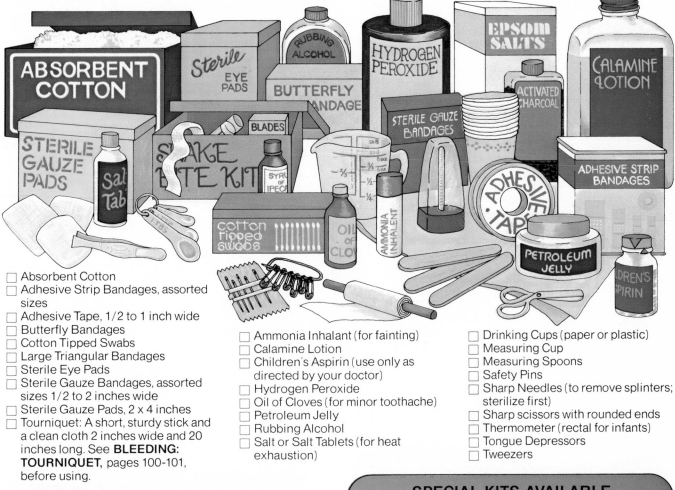

- [ ] Absorbent Cotton
- [ ] Adhesive Strip Bandages, assorted sizes
- [ ] Adhesive Tape, 1/2 to 1 inch wide
- [ ] Butterfly Bandages
- [ ] Cotton Tipped Swabs
- [ ] Large Triangular Bandages
- [ ] Sterile Eye Pads
- [ ] Sterile Gauze Bandages, assorted sizes 1/2 to 2 inches wide
- [ ] Sterile Gauze Pads, 2 x 4 inches
- [ ] Tourniquet: A short, sturdy stick and a clean cloth 2 inches wide and 20 inches long. See **BLEEDING: TOURNIQUET,** pages 100-101, before using.

- [ ] Ammonia Inhalant (for fainting)
- [ ] Calamine Lotion
- [ ] Children's Aspirin (use only as directed by your doctor)
- [ ] Hydrogen Peroxide
- [ ] Oil of Cloves (for minor toothache)
- [ ] Petroleum Jelly
- [ ] Rubbing Alcohol
- [ ] Salt or Salt Tablets (for heat exhaustion)

- [ ] Drinking Cups (paper or plastic)
- [ ] Measuring Cup
- [ ] Measuring Spoons
- [ ] Safety Pins
- [ ] Sharp Needles (to remove splinters; sterilize first)
- [ ] Sharp scissors with rounded ends
- [ ] Thermometer (rectal for infants)
- [ ] Tongue Depressors
- [ ] Tweezers

FOR ACCIDENTAL POISONING
- [ ] Syrup of Ipecac (to induce vomiting)
- [ ] Activated Charcoal (to absorb poison)
- [ ] Epsom Salts (a strong laxative; **use only as directed by your Poison Control Center)**
See **SWALLOWED POISONS,** page 181.

SPECIAL KITS AVAILABLE
Insect Sting Kit: For persons with severe allergic reactions. Available by prescription only.

Snake Bite Kit: Contains a constricting band, sterile blades and a suction device.

Poison First-Aid Kit: Contains syrup of ipecac, activated charcoal and Epsom salts.

Immunization Schedule

2 MONTHS	Combined Diphtheria-Tetanus-Pertussis (Whooping Cough): 1st shot Trivalent Oral Polio Vaccine: 1st dose
4 MONTHS	Combined Diphtheria-Tetanus-Pertussis: 2nd shot Trivalent Oral Polio Vaccine: 2nd dose
6 MONTHS	Combined Diphtheria-Tetanus-Pertussis: 3rd shot Trivalent Oral Polio Vaccine: 3rd dose
12 MONTHS	Tuberculin Test
15 MONTHS	Measles: may be given as combination Measles-Rubella or Measles-Mumps-Rubella
18 MONTHS	Combined Diphtheria-Tetanus-Pertussis: booster shot Trivalent Oral Polio Vaccine: booster dose
4 TO 6 YEARS	Combined Diphtheria-Tetanus-Pertussis: booster shot Trivalent Oral Polio Vaccine: booster dose
14 TO 16 YEARS	Combined Tetanus-Diphtheria: booster shot

• If there is a measles epidemic, the child should be given a measles shot even if he is not yet 15 months old.

• For deep punctures or severe wounds, a tetanus shot should be given immediately.

• Smallpox immunization is no longer routinely recommended.

• For foreign travel, follow your doctor's recommendations.

Immunization Record

NAME _____ DATE OF BIRTH _____

DIPHTHERIA-TETANUS-PERTUSSIS
1st DATE _____ PHYSICIAN _____
2nd DATE _____ PHYSICIAN _____
3rd DATE _____ PHYSICIAN _____
Booster DATE _____ PHYSICIAN _____
Booster DATE _____ PHYSICIAN _____

TRIVALENT ORAL POLIO VACCINE
1st DATE _____ PHYSICIAN _____
2nd DATE _____ PHYSICIAN _____
3rd DATE _____ PHYSICIAN _____
Booster DATE _____ PHYSICIAN _____
Booster DATE _____ PHYSICIAN _____

TUBERCULIN TEST
DATE _____ PHYSICIAN _____

MEASLES-MUMPS-RUBELLA
DATE _____ PHYSICIAN _____

TETANUS-DIPHTHERIA BOOSTER
DATE _____ PHYSICIAN _____

OTHER VACCINES (INFLUENZA, ETC.)
TYPE _____ DATE _____ PHYSICIAN _____
TYPE _____ DATE _____ PHYSICIAN _____
TYPE _____ DATE _____ PHYSICIAN _____
TYPE _____ DATE _____ PHYSICIAN _____
TYPE _____ DATE _____ PHYSICIAN _____

NAME _____ DATE OF BIRTH _____

DIPHTHERIA-TETANUS-PERTUSSIS
1st DATE _____ PHYSICIAN _____
2nd DATE _____ PHYSICIAN _____
3rd DATE _____ PHYSICIAN _____
Booster DATE _____ PHYSICIAN _____
Booster DATE _____ PHYSICIAN _____

TRIVALENT ORAL POLIO VACCINE
1st DATE _____ PHYSICIAN _____
2nd DATE _____ PHYSICIAN _____
3rd DATE _____ PHYSICIAN _____
Booster DATE _____ PHYSICIAN _____
Booster DATE _____ PHYSICIAN _____

TUBERCULIN TEST
DATE _____ PHYSICIAN _____

MEASLES-MUMPS-RUBELLA
DATE _____ PHYSICIAN _____

TETANUS-DIPHTHERIA BOOSTER
DATE _____ PHYSICIAN _____

OTHER VACCINES (INFLUENZA, ETC.)
TYPE _____ DATE _____ PHYSICIAN _____
TYPE _____ DATE _____ PHYSICIAN _____
TYPE _____ DATE _____ PHYSICIAN _____
TYPE _____ DATE _____ PHYSICIAN _____
TYPE _____ DATE _____ PHYSICIAN _____

NAME _____ DATE OF BIRTH _____

DIPHTHERIA-TETANUS-PERTUSSIS
1st DATE _____ PHYSICIAN _____
2nd DATE _____ PHYSICIAN _____
3rd DATE _____ PHYSICIAN _____
Booster DATE _____ PHYSICIAN _____
Booster DATE _____ PHYSICIAN _____

TRIVALENT ORAL POLIO VACCINE
1st DATE _____ PHYSICIAN _____
2nd DATE _____ PHYSICIAN _____
3rd DATE _____ PHYSICIAN _____
Booster DATE _____ PHYSICIAN _____
Booster DATE _____ PHYSICIAN _____

TUBERCULIN TEST
DATE _____ PHYSICIAN _____

MEASLES-MUMPS-RUBELLA
DATE _____ PHYSICIAN _____

TETANUS-DIPHTHERIA BOOSTER
DATE _____ PHYSICIAN _____

OTHER VACCINES (INFLUENZA, ETC.)
TYPE _____ DATE _____ PHYSICIAN _____
TYPE _____ DATE _____ PHYSICIAN _____
TYPE _____ DATE _____ PHYSICIAN _____
TYPE _____ DATE _____ PHYSICIAN _____
TYPE _____ DATE _____ PHYSICIAN _____

Childhood Illnesses

	SYMPTOMS	INCUBATION	DURATION
BRONCHITIS	Frequent coughing. Labored breathing. Possible fever.	1 to 7 days	2 to 4 days
CHICKEN POX	Fever. Discomfort. Itching. Pink or red spots on the chest, stomach and back, which may spread to the scalp and face. Spots change to blisters, which eventually crust.	10 to 21 days	7 to 10 days
COMMON COLD	Sneezing. Stuffed or runny nose. Sore throat. Watery eyes. Possible cough, chills, low fever.	1 to 7 days	2 to 14 days
CROUP	Labored breathing. Hoarseness. Loud hacking cough. Often comes on at night.	2 to 6 days	4 to 5 days
GERMAN MEASLES (RUBELLA)	Chills. Low fever (sometimes high). Runny nose. Painful swelling of glands behind the ears. Usually there is a slightly raised fine red rash, which begins on the face, then spreads over the entire body.	14 to 21 days	3 to 6 days
INFLUENZA (VIRUS, FLU)	Chills. Drowsiness. Weakness. Sudden high fever. Headache. Achiness. Sore throat. No appetite. Possible nausea and dizziness.	1 to 3 days	3 to 7 days
MEASLES	Early symptoms include low fever, slight hacking cough, fatigue, discomfort, eye irritation. Around the 4th day, fever and cough worsen and a rash of faint pink spots appears on the neck and cheeks, then spreads to the rest of the body.	10 to 15 days	8 to 12 days
MUMPS	Swollen glands on one or both sides of the jaw. Mild headache. Fever.	12 to 24 days	6 to 10 days
PNEUMONIA	Coughing. Fever. Rapid breathing. Discomfort. Chills. Weakness. Possible nausea and vomiting. Sudden fever lasting several days.	2 to 14 days	About 7 days
ROSEOLA	Sudden fever lasting several days. After fever is gone, a rash of flat or raised spots appears on the chest, stomach or back, then spreads to the rest of the body.	10 to 14 days	5 to 6 days
SCARLET FEVER	Painful sore throat. Fever. Nausea and vomiting. Within 3 days a fine rash appears on the neck, armpit and groin, then spreads over the body.	1 to 5 days	6 to 8 days
STREP THROAT	Painful sore throat. Fever. Nausea and vomiting.	2 to 5 days	About 6 days

VOMITING AND DIARRHEA

Consult your doctor if vomiting or diarrhea persists for more than 6 hours, contains blood or is accompanied by high fever. Have the child rest and keep him off solid foods. When he starts to feel better, give him low fat foods and frequent small amounts of liquid.

COMMUNICABILITY	TREATMENT*	SPECIAL PRECAUTIONS
2 days before symptoms appear to 2 days after	**Consult your doctor.** If the child has fever, make sure he rests, give him plenty of juice and use a vaporizer.	
1 day before spots appear to about 6 days after. The child should be isolated until blisters crust and dry.	**Consult your doctor.** Rest is essential. Relieve itching with calamine lotion. Trim the child's nails so he doesn't scratch himself.	Keep his utensils and dishes separate.
2 days before symptoms appear to 2 days after	If the child has fever, make sure he rests, give him plenty of juice and use a vaporizer. Keep him warm and avoid chilling.	Consult your doctor if the symptoms persist or worsen.
2 days before symptoms appear to 5 days after	**Consult your doctor.** Use a vaporizer. Keep the child on a light, low fat diet.	
7 days before symptoms appear to 5 days after. **Pregnant women should never be exposed to this illness.**	If the child has fever, make sure he rests, give him plenty of juice and use a vaporizer.	Keep the child's hands clean. Launder his linen and clothes separately.
1 day before symptoms appear to 7 days after	**Consult your doctor.** If the child has fever, make sure he rests, give him plenty of juice and use a vaporizer.	Keep his utensils and dishes separate.
4 days before rash appears to 5 days after	**Consult your doctor.** If the child's eyes are sensitive to light, keep the room dim. If he has fever, make sure he rests, give him plenty of juice and use a vaporizer.	Keep his utensils and dishes separate.
7 days before symptoms appear to 9 days after	**Consult your doctor.** Rest is essential. Apply cool compresses to the cheeks. **Do not** give the child citrus juices.	Keep his utensils and dishes separate.
Varies	**Consult your doctor.** Make sure the child rests. Give him plenty of juice. Use a vaporizer. Keep him on a light, low fat diet.	
Varies	**Consult your doctor.**	
1 day before symptoms appear to 6 days after	**Consult your doctor.** Make sure the child rests. Give him plenty of fluids.	Check other family members for symptoms.
1 day before symptoms appear to 6 days after	**Consult your doctor.** If the child has fever, make sure he rests and give him plenty of juice.	Check other family members for symptoms.

* If a fever reaches 103°F. (39.46°C.), see **FEVER**, pages 156-157.

IMPORTANT: Watch breathing closely. If it stops, see **BREATHING: ARTIFICIAL RESPIRATION,** pages 124-127.

For any drug overdose, call your local Poison Control Center immediately. Also seek medical aid.

For ingested drugs, induce vomiting if the child is conscious. See **SWALLOWED POISONS,** page 181, and follow treatment **B**.

Do not panic or threaten a child intoxicated by a drug. Be supportive, tolerant and gentle.

Keep the environment quiet and peaceful if the drug is being well tolerated. The effects will gradually wear off.

DRUG IDENTIFICATION

SEDATIVES

EFFECTS OF HABITUAL USE MAY INCLUDE: Sleepiness. Slurred speech. Irritability. Lack of coordination. Confused thinking. Dulled reactions. Impaired memory. Coma.
When taken with alcohol, may be fatal.

BARBITURATES
(Amytal, Nembutal, Phenobarbital, Seconal, Tuinal, Etc.)

Amytal   Nembutal   Seconal   Tuinal

IMPORTANT: Barbiturates are highly addictive.
Duration: 4 to 8 hours

HYPNOTICS
(Doriden, Quaalude, Sopor, Etc.)

Doriden   Quaalude   Sopor

Duration: 4 to 8 hours

TRANQUILIZERS
(Equanil, Librium, Miltown, Placidyl, Valium, Etc.)

Equanil   Librium   Miltown   Placidyl   Valium

Duration: 2 to 8 hours

TREATMENT FOR AN OVERDOSE
- **Seek medical aid immediately.**
- If the child has trouble breathing, see **BREATHING: ARTIFICIAL RESPIRATION,** pages 124-127.
- Treat for **SHOCK,** pages 188-189.
- A heavily addicted user should not try to withdraw abruptly.

STIMULANTS

EFFECTS MAY INCLUDE: Elation. Loss of appetite. Increased energy and alertness. **Frequent large doses can produce** trembling, muscle spasms, deep depression, hallucinations, convulsions and coma.

AMPHETAMINES
(Benzedrine, Biphetamine, Desoxyn, Dexamyl, Dexedrine, Methamphetamine, Preludin, Ritalin, Etc.)

Benzedrine   Biphetamine

Desoxyn   Dexamyl

Dexedrine   Methamphetamine

Crystal

Preludin   Ritalin

Further effects can include incessant talking, insomnia, irritability and restlessness, impaired judgment, malnutrition and extreme weight loss, and paranoia.
Duration: 3 to 4 hours.

COCAINE

Further effects can include impaired nasal membranes.
Duration: 15 to 30 minutes

TREATMENT FOR AN OVERDOSE
Seek medical aid and give supportive care.

OPIATES (NARCOTICS)

IMPORTANT: All opiates are highly addictive.
EFFECTS MAY INCLUDE: Tranquil, euphoric feeling. Dizziness, nausea and vomiting. Itchiness. Sweating. Constipation. Loss of appetite and physical energy. Very small pupils. Disassociation. Sluggishness. Drowsiness. Slurred speech. Slow pulse and respiration. Lowered temperature. Weight loss and overall breakdown in health.

HEROIN

Duration: 4 to 6 hours

MORPHINE

Duration: May last 12 hours or more

METHADONE

Duration: 4 to 6 hours

OPIUM

Duration: 2 to 6 hours

OTHER OPIUM DERIVATIVES
(Codeine, Demerol, Dilaudid, Paregoric, Etc.)

Codeine   **Demerol**   **Dilaudid**   **Paregoric**

Duration: 2 to 8 hours

TREATMENT FOR AN OVERDOSE
- **Seek medical aid immediately.**
- If the child has trouble breathing, see **BREATHING: ARTIFICIAL RESPIRATION,** pages 124-127.
- If he has trouble staying conscious, arouse him. Keep him awake and moving constantly.
- Treat for **SHOCK,** pages 188-189.
- Keep calm. Stay with the child, giving him emotional support and gentle reassurance.

HALLUCINOGENS

EFFECTS: Vary greatly according to the individual, the dose, the potency and the circumstances. Experiences can be highly pleasurable or frightening and bizarre. Psychotic reactions can be provoked in susceptible persons. Effects may include: Intense visual imagery. Intensification of the senses. Feelings of deep, spiritual transcendence. Distortion of time and space. Hallucinations. Dizziness and nausea. Numbness. Poor coordination. Panic, fear and depression.

LSD (Lysergic Acid Diethylamide)

Duration: Varies with dose, potency and user.
Usually 6 to 18 hours

MESCALINE

Duration: 6 to 12 hours

PEYOTE BUTTONS

Duration: 6 to 12 hours

PSILOCYBIN

Duration: 5 to 8 hours

TREATMENT FOR AN ADVERSE REACTION
- **Seek medical aid** if the child becomes panicky, violent or severely depressed.
- Protect him from hurting himself.
- Give him emotional support and gentle reassurance. **Do not** frighten or berate him.

71

CANNABIS (Marijuana, Hashish)

EFFECTS MAY INCLUDE: Reddened eyes. Intensification of mood, feelings and senses. Lessening of anxieties and inhibitions. Increased appetite, particularly for sweets. Distortion of time and space. Euphoria. Lightheadedness. Irritability and nervousness. Fear and paranoia.

Hashish

Marijuana

Duration: 30 minutes to several hours

TREATMENT FOR AN ADVERSE REACTION

- Give the child emotional support and gentle reassurance. **Do not** frighten or berate him.
- **Seek medical aid** if the child becomes panicky, violent or severely depressed.

ALCOHOL

IMPORTANT: Alcohol is highly addictive.

EFFECTS MAY INCLUDE: Drowsiness. Slurred speech. Dizziness, nausea and vomiting. Lack of coordination. Uninhibited behavior. Impaired reactions and judgment. Aggressiveness. Loss of consciousness. Habitual use can damage the liver, brain, nervous system and heart.

ONE QUART
GIN

ONE QUART
Whiskey

Wine

INHALANTS (Aerosols, Airplane Glue, Etc.)

EFFECTS MAY INCLUDE: Slurred speech. Impaired reactions and judgment. Mild euphoria. Lack of coordination. Hallucinations. Rapid pulse. Habitual use can damage the liver, kidneys and brain.

TREATMENT FOR AN OVERDOSE
- **Seek medical aid immediately.**
- If the child has trouble breathing, see **BREATHING: ARTIFICIAL RESPIRATION**, pages 124-127.
- Treat for **SHOCK**, pages 188-189.

SPRAY
Plastic Coating

Airplane Glue

Duration: Varies with dosage.

ASPIRIN

TREATMENT FOR AN OVERDOSE
Call your local Poison Control Center and seek immediate medical aid. See **SWALLOWED POISONS,** page 181, and follow treatment **B**.

PART TWO

Emergencies
First-Aid Procedures

IMPORTANT: If the injury seems at all serious, **send for medical aid immediately.**

Do not move the child unless absolutely necessary. You may cause further harm.

Remain calm and offer reassurance and comfort.

Check the child for emergency medical information tags or cards.

1 **Check the pulse** (below the left nipple for an infant; at the large artery of the neck for an older child). If no pulse is felt, see **HEART FAILURE,** pages 170-173.

2 **Check the child's breathing.** If necessary, see **BREATHING: ARTIFICIAL RESPIRATION,** pages 124-127.

3 **Check for bleeding.** Quickly and gently examine the child's head and body for injuries. Make sure not to overlook any concealed wounds. Control the most serious bleeding first. See **BLEEDING,** pages 96-97.

4 If there are burns or stains on the child's mouth or other signs of poisoning (pills, chemicals, etc.), see **POISONING,** pages 180-187.

5 If the child is seriously injured, treat for **SHOCK,** pages 188-189.

6 For broken bones, see **BREAKS, FRACTURES & DISLOCATIONS,** pages 112-123.

7 In cool or cold weather, particularly if it is windy and the child is wet, see **COLD EXPOSURE: HYPOTHERMIA,** pages 160-161.

QUICK REFERENCE

ASSESSING THE EMERGENCY

- Check The Pulse
- Check Breathing
- Check For Bleeding
- Check For Poisoning
- Check For Shock
- Check For Broken Bones

BACK & NECK INJURIES
86-87

BITES & STINGS
88-95

ANIMAL & HUMAN BITES p.88

INSECTS p.90

MARINE LIFE p.92

SNAKE BITE p.94

POISONOUS SNAKE

NONPOISONOUS SNAKE

76

QUICK REFERENCE

BLEEDING: CUTS & WOUNDS
Pages **96-111**

DIRECT PRESSURE p.96

PRESSURE POINTS p.98

TOURNIQUET p.100

IMPALED OBJECTS p.106

FISHHOOKS p.108

INTERNAL BLEEDING p.104

AMPUTATIONS p.110

BREAKS: FRACTURES & DISLOCATIONS
112-123

COLLARBONE & SHOULDER p.112

BENT ELBOW p.112

STRAIGHT ELBOW p.114

FINGERS p.114

ARM, WRIST & HAND p.116

PELVIS & HIP p.118

KNEE p.120

LEG & ANKLE p.120

FOOT & TOES p.122

QUICK REFERENCE

BREATHING: ARTIFICIAL RESPIRATION
Pages **124-127**

INFANT & SMALL CHILD p.124

OLDER CHILD p.126

BURNS
128-133

CHEMICAL p.128

1st & 2nd DEGREE p.130

3rd DEGREE p.132

CHEST INJURIES
134-139

CRUSHED CHEST p.134

OPEN CHEST WOUNDS p.136

RIBS p.138

CHOKING
140-141

QUICK REFERENCE

CONVULSIONS & SEIZURES Pages **142-143**

DROWNING **144-147**

WATER RESCUE p.144

ICE RESCUE p.146

EAR INJURIES **148-149**

FOREIGN OBJECTS

EMERGENCY ROOM

CUTS

ELECTRIC SHOCK **150-151**

FUSE

QUICK REFERENCE

EYE INJURIES
Pages 152-155

FOREIGN OBJECTS p.152   **CHEMICALS p.152**   **LACERATED EYEBALL p.154**   **IMPALED OBJECTS p.154**

FEVER
156-157

FROSTBITE & COLD EXPOSURE
158-161

FROSTBITE p.158

COLD EXPOSURE: HYPOTHERMIA p.160

QUICK REFERENCE

HEAD INJURIES
Pages 162-169

CLOSED p.162   OPEN p.164   SKULL & CHEEK p.166   FACE & JAW p.168

HEART FAILURE
170-173

INFANT & SMALL CHILD p.170   OLDER CHILD p.172

HEART ATTACK
174-175

MOUTH INJURIES
176-177

GUMS & PALATE   TEETH   LIPS   TONGUE

QUICK REFERENCE

NOSE INJURIES

Pages **178-179**

NOSE BLEED

BROKEN NOSE

POISONING

180-187

SWALLOWED p.180

INHALED p.182

PLANTS p.186

SHOCK

188-189

SPRAINS & STRAINS

190-191

SPRAINS

STRAINS

STOMACH INJURIES

Pages 192-193

SUNSTROKE & HEAT EXHAUSTION

194-195

SUNSTROKE

HEAT EXHAUSTION

TRANSPORTING THE INJURED

196-199

NECK & SPINE INJURIES p.196

STRETCHERS p.198

CARRIES p.199

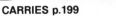

83

For all serious emergencies, first check:

- **BREATHING**
- Pulse **(HEART FAILURE)**
- **BLEEDING**
- **SHOCK**

If in doubt about the injury, see:
ASSESSING THE EMERGENCY, pages 74-75

1 Place your thumb on the appropriate emergency tab.

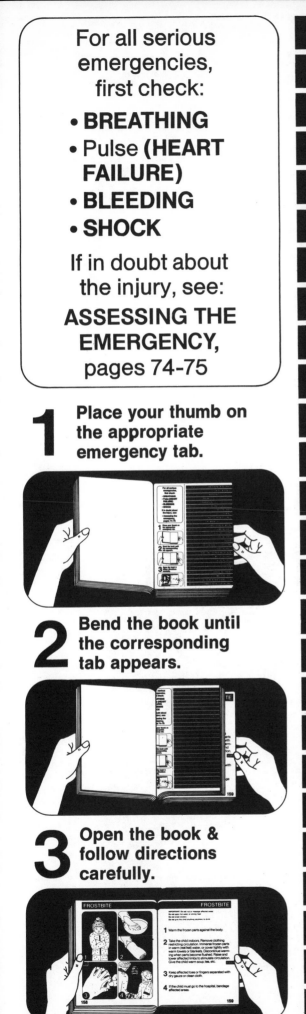

2 Bend the book until the corresponding tab appears.

3 Open the book & follow directions carefully.

BACK & NECK INJURIES

1A

1B

2

IMPORTANT: **Seek medical aid immediately.**

Do not bend or twist the neck or body.

Do not move the child unless you absolutely must. If it does become necessary, see **TRANSPORTING THE INJURED,** pages 196-197.

If the child has trouble breathing, see **BREATHING: ARTIFICIAL RESPIRATION,** pages 124-127.

1A Immobilize the head in the position found by placing rolled up clothing, blankets, etc. around the head and the sides of the neck and shoulders. For back injuries, also immobilize the torso.

1B If the child is on her back, slide a small towel or pad under her neck without moving her head. (**Do not** place anything bulky under the head.)

2 Hold restraining materials in place with bricks, stones, etc.

BITES & STINGS:

IMPORTANT: If the skin is penetrated, seek medical aid immediately. Human bites can be particularly dangerous.
Try to capture or confine the animal for examination.
Observe for **SHOCK,** pages 188-189.

1 Control the bleeding. See **BLEEDING,** pages 96-97.

2 Wash the wound with soap and water. **Do not** use antiseptics, ointments or other medications.

3 Apply a sterile dressing or clean cloth, and hold it in place with a bandage.

BITES & STINGS: INSECTS

IMPORTANT: Seek medical aid immediately for bites and stings from **BLACK WIDOW** and **BROWN RECLUSE SPIDERS, SCORPIONS** and **TARANTULAS,** particularly if the child is subject to hay fever, asthma or an allergic reaction. Also observe for **SHOCK,** pages 188-189.

BEDBUG

SYMPTOMS: Welts. Swelling. Irritation.

FIRST AID: Wash thoroughly with soap and water.

BEE (WASP, HORNET & YELLOW JACKET)

NOTE: Seek medical aid immediately if the child is subject to allergic reactions or if there is severe swelling anywhere on his body. Also observe for **SHOCK,** pages 188-189, and watch breathing closely. If necessary, see **BREATHING: ARTIFICIAL RESPIRATION,** pages 124-127.

SYMPTOMS: Pain. Local swelling. Burning and itching. Allergic reaction will also cause nausea, shock, unconsciousness and severe swelling.

FIRST AID: For a bee sting, remove the venom sac by scraping gently, not by squeezing. (Wasps, hornets and yellow jackets do not leave venom sacs.) Wash with soap and water. For severe reactions, see first aid for **BLACK WIDOW.**

BLACK WIDOW SPIDER

SYMPTOMS: Severe pain. Profuse sweating. Muscle cramps. Difficulty breathing. Nausea.

FIRST AID: Watch breathing closely. If it stops, see **BREATHING: ARTIFICIAL RESPIRATION,** pages 124-127. Keep the child quiet and avoid unnecessary movement. Keep the affected part below heart level. Place a constricting band 2 to 4 inches above the wound. **Do not** bind too tightly. You should be able to slide your finger under it. Apply ice wrapped in a cloth. Remove the band after 30 minutes.

BITES & STINGS: INSECTS

BROWN RECLUSE SPIDER

SYMPTOMS: The bite may be hardly noticed, but hours later severe pain, swelling and blisters occur.

FIRST AID: Follow first aid for **BLACK WIDOW.**

CHIGGER

SYMPTOMS: Itching. Irritation. Local pain. Small red welts.

FIRST AID: Wash with soap and water. Soothe irritation with cold compresses or calamine lotion.

MOSQUITO

SYMPTOMS: Itching. Irritation. Local pain. Small red welts.

FIRST AID: Wash with soap and water. Soothe irritation with cold compresses or calamine lotion.

SCORPION

SYMPTOMS: Excruciating pain at the sting. Swelling. Fever. Nausea. Stomach pains. Difficulty speaking. Worsening convulsions. Coma.

FIRST AID: Follow first aid for **BLACK WIDOW.**

TARANTULA

SYMPTOMS: May vary from pin prick to severe wound.

FIRST AID: Wash with soap and water. Cover lightly with a sterile dressing or clean cloth. For severe reactions, see first aid for **BLACK WIDOW.**

TICK

SYMPTOMS: The tick may be visible on the skin as a dark spot.

FIRST AID: Do not pull the tick from the child's skin. Apply heavy oil to the area, then after 30 minutes remove the parts carefully with a tweezer. Wash with soap and water.

IMPORTANT: Seek medical aid immediately.
Watch breathing closely. If necessary, see **BREATHING: ARTIFICIAL RESPIRATION,** pages 124-127.
Observe for **SHOCK,** pages 188-189.

CONE SHELL

SYMPTOMS: Vary from a slight sting to severe pain, numbness, tingling, difficulty swallowing, tightness in the chest, partial paralysis, impaired vision, collapse.

FIRST AID: Place a constricting band 2 to 4 inches above the wound. **Do not** bind too tightly. You should be able to slide your finger under it. Soak in hot water or apply hot compresses for 30 minutes, then remove the band.

MAN OF WAR & JELLYFISH

SYMPTOMS: Burning pain. Rash. Swelling. Difficulty breathing. Cramps. Nausea. Vomiting. Collapse.

FIRST AID: Gently remove the tentacles with a cloth. Clean affected area with alcohol or diluted ammonia.

SEA ANEMONE & HYDROID

SYMPTOMS: Burning or stinging pain. Stomach cramps. Chills. Diarrhea.

FIRST AID: Soak in hot water or apply hot compresses.

SEA URCHIN

SYMPTOMS: Pain. Dizziness. Muscle tremors. Paralysis.

FIRST AID: Follow first aid for **CONE SHELL.**

STINGING CORAL

SYMPTOMS: Burning or stinging pain.

FIRST AID: Wash thoroughly with soap and water.

STINGRAY

SYMPTOMS: Painful cut or puncture. Swelling. Discoloration. Nausea. Vomiting. Muscle spasms. Convulsions. Difficulty breathing.

FIRST AID: Carefully remove the stinger if possible. Wash thoroughly with soap and water. Control the bleeding; see **BLEED-ING,** pages 96-97. Apply a constricting band; see first aid for **CONE SHELL.**

BITES & STINGS: SNAKE BITE

IMPORTANT: To determine if the bite is from a poisonous snake, look for fang marks at the wound. If nonpoisonous, see Step 4 only.

Send for medical aid immediately.

Do not let the child walk or move the affected part unless absolutely necessary.

Watch breathing closely. If necessary, see **BREATHING: ARTIFICIAL RESPIRATION,** pages 124-127.

Treat for **SHOCK,** pages 188-189.

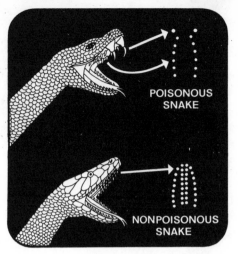

POISONOUS SNAKE

NONPOISONOUS SNAKE

SYMPTOMS: Vary from slight burning and mild swelling to acute pain and severe swelling. Can include nausea, vomiting, difficulty breathing, dim or blurred vision, weakness, slurred speech, sweating, paralysis, convulsions.

1 Apply a constricting band between the bite and the heart 2 to 4 inches above the puncture. **Do not** bind too tightly. Check the pulse below the wound. If you can't feel it, loosen the band until it returns. The wound should ooze. Keep the affected part below heart level.

2 Clean the wound with alcohol. Sterilize a knife or razor blade over an open flame, and make a **shallow vertical incision 1/2 inch long over each fang mark. Do not** cut deeply or crisscross.

3 Draw the venom from the wound with a suction cup or your mouth, if it is free of open sores. **Do not** swallow the venom. Maintain suction for 30 minutes. If swelling reaches the band, leave it in place and apply a second band 2 to 4 inches above the first.

4 Wash thoroughly with soap and water. Apply cold compresses or ice wrapped in a cloth. **Do not** pack in ice.

1

2

3

4

IMPORTANT: Seek medical aid for any serious bleeding.
Do not apply direct pressure on breaks.
Observe for **SHOCK,** pages 188-189.

First try to control the bleeding by **DIRECT PRESSURE**; see below.
If you cannot control the bleeding, use **PRESSURE POINTS,**
pages 98-99, while continuing **DIRECT PRESSURE.**
If serious blood loss continues and becomes critical, apply
a **TOURNIQUET** as a last resort; see pages 100-103.

1 Press gauze or a clean cloth directly over the wound.

2 Elevate injured limbs higher than the heart unless there is evidence of fracture.

3 After bleeding is controlled, bandage firmly but not too tightly.

4 Check the pulse below the wound. If you can't feel it, loosen the bandage until it returns, then treat for **SHOCK,** pages 188-189.

98

IMPORTANT: Seek medical aid for any serious bleeding.
Continue **DIRECT PRESSURE,** pages 96-97, and elevate the wound.
Observe for **SHOCK,** pages 188-189.

A **Scalp:** Press your thumb against the bone just in front of the child's ear.

B **Face:** Press your fingers against the hollow spot in the jaw.

C **Neck:** Place your thumb against the back of the child's neck. Put your fingers on the side of the neck just before (not over) the windpipe, and press toward your thumb.

D **Chest or Armpit:** Press your thumb in the groove behind the child's collarbone.

E **Arm:** Place your fingers on the inner side of the arm, pressing in the groove between the muscles. Keeping your thumb on the outside of the arm, press toward the bone.

F **Hand:** Place your thumb on the inner side of the wrist and press toward the bone.

G **Leg:** Place the heel of your hand on the inner thigh at the crease of the groin. Press against the bone.

BLEEDING: CUTS & WOUNDS

TOURNIQUET

1

2

3

**IMPORTANT: Seek medical aid immediately.
Do not use except in a critical emergency where all other methods
fail and it's a matter of life over limb.** First try **DIRECT PRESSURE,**
pages 96-97, and **PRESSURE POINTS,** pages 98-99.
The tourniquet band must be at least 2 inches wide.

1 Place the tourniquet band over the artery to
be compressed, **slightly above** the wound.
If a joint intervenes, position the band above
the joint.

2 Wrap the band tightly around the limb twice,
and tie a half knot.

3 Place a short, strong stick on the band, and
complete the knot on the top of the stick.

CONTINUED ON NEXT PAGE

4

5

6

102

4 Twist the stick until the bleeding stops.

5 Secure the stick in place. **Do not** loosen unless a doctor so advises.

6 Write down the exact time the tourniquet was applied. Attach it as a note to the child's clothes or write it on his forehead with lipstick, etc. Treat for **SHOCK,** pages 188-189, and get to the hospital immediately.

IMPORTANT: To be suspected if the child has had a sharp blow or crushing injury to the abdomen, chest or torso.
Do not give the child anything to drink.
Seek medical aid.

SYMPTOMS: Stomach: Vomit is bright red, dark red or the color and size of large coffee grounds.
Intestines: Excrement contains dark tar-like material or bright red blood.
Chest and Lungs: Bright red foamy blood is coughed up.

1 Keep the child lying down and covered lightly. Turn the head to one side to keep the air passage clear.

2 Raise her head if she has difficulty breathing.

BLEEDING: CUTS & WOUNDS

IMPALED OBJECTS

IMPORTANT: Call for an ambulance or get to the hospital immediately.
Do not move the child off an impaling object unless his life is in imminent danger. If you must, remove him as gently as possible, tend to his wounds immediately, and treat for **SHOCK,** pages 188-189.

1 If possible, cut off the impaling object several inches from the wound without moving or removing it.

2 Carefully cut away the clothing from around the wound.

3 Place bulky dressings around the object.

4 Secure the dressings in place with bandages. Treat for **SHOCK,** pages 188-189.

BLEEDING: CUTS & WOUNDS FISHHOOKS

108

BLEEDING: CUTS & WOUNDS FISHHOOKS

IMPORTANT: Do not attempt to remove a fishhook from the child's face. **Seek medical aid immediately.**

1 Push the shank through the skin until the point appears.

2 Cut off the barbed end with clippers or pliers.

3 Remove the shank from the wound.

4 Wash the wound with soap and water. Cover with gauze or a clean cloth. **Consult your doctor.**

110

IMPORTANT: Stay calm and act quickly. Bleeding must be stopped as soon as possible.
Seek medical aid immediately.

1 Control the bleeding through **DIRECT PRESSURE,** pages 96-97, and **PRESSURE POINTS,** pages 98-99. As a last resort, a **TOURNIQUET** may be necessary, pages 100-103.

2 Treat for **SHOCK,** pages 188-189.

3 Wrap severed parts in a cold, wet dressing, then place in a plastic bag and pack in ice. Transport to the hospital with the child.

BREAKS: FRACTURES & DISLOCATIONS

COLLARBONE, SHOULDER & BENT ELBOW

COLLARBONE & SHOULDER

1

2

BENT ELBOW

1

2

IMPORTANT: Seek medical aid.
Do not try to reset dislocations yourself.
Treat the same as fractures.
If any bones protrude, control the bleeding and cover the wound
with a large clean dressing or cloth. **Do not** clean the wound.
Observe for **SHOCK,** pages 188-189.

BREAKS: COLLARBONE, SHOULDER & BENT ELBOW

COLLARBONE & SHOULDER

1 Make a sling to support the weight of the arm.

2 Immobilize the arm by tying a band over the sling and around the body.

BENT ELBOW

1 Immobilize in the position found with a padded splint. Use boards, magazines, etc. for rigidity; cloth for padding.

2 Make a sling to support the weight of the arm, and bind it to the body. Be sure the fingers are above elbow level.

BREAKS: FRACTURES & DISLOCATIONS

STRAIGHT ELBOW & FINGERS

STRAIGHT ELBOW

FINGERS

114

IMPORTANT: Seek medical aid.
Do not try to reset dislocations yourself.
Treat the same as fractures.
If any bones protrude, control the bleeding and cover the wound with a large clean dressing or cloth. **Do not** clean the wound.
Observe for **SHOCK,** pages 188-189.

STRAIGHT ELBOW

1 Immobilize the elbow in position with a padded splint extending from the armpit to the hand. Use boards, magazines, etc. for rigidity; cloth for padding.

FINGERS

1 Make a padded splint out of a tongue depressor or the like.

2 Bind it to the finger with cloth or tape.

BREAKS: ARM, WRIST & HAND

1

2

3

4

116

BREAKS: ARM, WRIST & HAND

IMPORTANT: Seek medical aid.
Do not try to reset dislocations yourself.
Treat the same as fractures.
Observe for **SHOCK,** pages 188-189.

1 If any bones protrude, control the bleeding and cover with a large clean dressing or cloth. **Do not** clean the wound.

2 Immobilize with a padded splint. Use boards, magazines, etc. for rigidity; cloth for padding. **Do not** tie too tightly.

3 Make a sling to support the weight of the arm. Be sure the fingers are above elbow level.

4 For a broken arm, immobilize the shoulder and elbow by binding the arm to the body.

1

2

118

IMPORTANT: Seek medical aid.
Observe for **SHOCK,** pages 188-189.

1 Check for fracture by gently feeling the bones in the pelvic and hip areas. Note where it hurts the child when you touch him.

2 To immobilize the child, place thick padding between his thighs, then tie him down on a board, door, etc. with bandages, belts or the like.

KNEE

LEG & ANKLE

IMPORTANT: Seek medical aid.
Do not try to reset dislocations yourself.
Treat the same as fractures.
Observe for **SHOCK,** pages 188-189.

BREAKS: KNEE, LEG & ANKLE

KNEE

1A Immobilize in the position found with a padded splint. Use boards, magazines, etc. for rigidity; cloth for padding.

1B For a straight knee, extend the splint from the buttock to the heel.

LEG & ANKLE

1 If any bones protrude, control the bleeding and cover with a large clean dressing or cloth. **Do not** clean the wound.

2A Immobilize with a padded splint. Use boards, magazines, etc. for rigidity; cloth or a pillow for padding.

2B If unable to improvise a splint, place padding between the legs and tie them together.

1

2

BREAKS: FOOT & TOES

IMPORTANT: Seek medical aid.
Do not try to reset dislocations yourself.
Treat the same as fractures.
Observe for **SHOCK,** pages 188-189.

1 Remove or cut away the shoe or boot if possible.

2 Immobilize with a padded splint. Tie it snugly but not too tightly. Use a blanket, pillow, etc.

BREATHING: INFANT & SMALL CHILD

1

2

3

IMPORTANT: Seek medical aid as quickly as possible.
Before beginning artificial respiration, quickly check
the pulse under the left nipple. If you cannot feel it, turn to
HEART FAILURE, pages 170-171.
Do not tip back the head if there is a neck or back injury.
To open the air passage, gently pull open the jaw without
moving the head.

1 Place the child on his back. If there is no neck or back injury, open the air passage by gently tipping back his head. If necessary, clear out his mouth with your fingers or a cloth. Re-check the pulse.

2 If breathing does not resume, place your open mouth over the child's nose and mouth, forming an airtight seal. Give 4 quick, gentle breaths.

3 Then give the child a new breath every 3 seconds, 20 per minute, using short gentle puffs of air. Remove your mouth between breaths and look and listen for the air leaving his lungs. If the entry or return of air seem blocked or the chest does not move, see **CHOKING,** pages 140-141, then resume artificial respiration at Step 1. Continue until the child breathes spontaneously. Treat for **SHOCK,** pages 188-189.

BREATHING: ARTIFICIAL RESPIRATION

OLDER CHILD

IMPORTANT: Seek medical aid as quickly as possible.
Before beginning artificial respiration, quickly check the pulse at the large artery in the neck. If you cannot feel it, turn to **HEART FAILURE,** pages 172-173.
Do not tip back the head if there is a neck or back injury. To open the air passage, gently pull open the jaw without moving the head.

1 Place the child on her back. If there is no neck or back injury, open the air passage by gently tipping back her head. If necessary, clear out her mouth with your fingers or a cloth. Re-check the pulse.

2 If breathing does not resume, open her jaws and pinch her nose closed. Place your mouth over her mouth, forming an airtight seal. Give 4 quick, gentle breaths.

3 Then give the child a new breath every 5 seconds, 12 per minute. Remove your mouth between breaths and look and listen for the air leaving her lungs. If the entry or return of air seems blocked or the chest does not move, see **CHOKING,** pages 140-141, then resume artificial respiration at Step 1. Continue until the child breathes spontaneously. Treat for **SHOCK,** pages 188-189.

BURNS: CHEMICAL

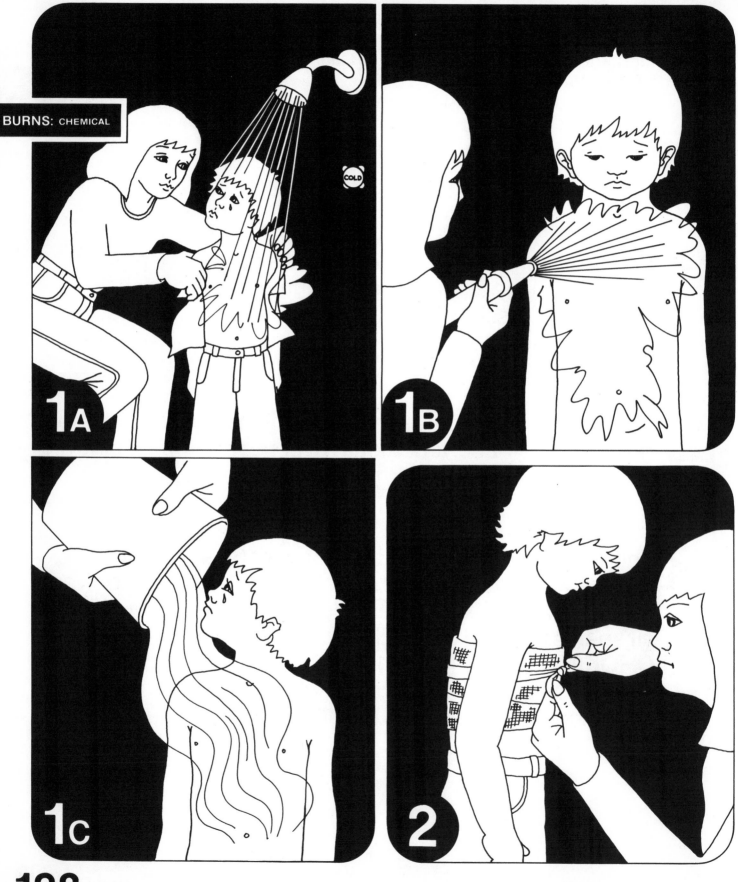

COLD

1A

1B

1C

2

128

IMPORTANT: Seek medical aid as soon as possible.

1A Place the child under a heavy, cool shower immediately. Remove all contaminated clothing. Keep him there at least 5 minutes, until all traces of the chemical have washed away.

1B If a shower is not available, use a hose.

1C If a hose isn't available, keep pouring cool water over the burn.

2 Cover with a clean, nonadhering dressing or cloth. Treat for **SHOCK,** pages 188-189.

BURNS: HEAT 1st & 2nd DEGREE

1A

1B

2

3

130

IMPORTANT: Do not remove shreds of tissue or break blisters.
Do not use antiseptic sprays, ointments or home remedies.
Do not put pressure on burned areas.
Observe for **SHOCK,** pages 188-189.
Seek medical aid.

Determine the degree of the burn and treat accordingly:
First Degree: Red or discolored skin. **See below.**
Second Degree: Blisters and red or mottled skin. **See below.**
Third Degree: White or charred skin. **See next page.**

1A Immerse in cold (**not ice**) water until pain subsides.

1B Or lightly apply cold clean compresses that have been wrung out in ice water.

2 Gently blot dry with sterile gauze or a clean cloth.

3 Cover loosely with a dry clean dressing. Elevate burned arms or legs higher than the heart.

BURNS: HEAT 3rd DEGREE

132

BURNS: HEAT 3rd DEGREE

IMPORTANT: Call for an ambulance or doctor immediately.

Do not apply water, antiseptic sprays, ointments or home remedies.

Do not remove adhered particles of clothing.

Do not remove shreds of tissue or break blisters.

Do not use absorbent cotton.

1 Lightly cover burned area with a nonadhering dressing or a dry, clean sheet or cloth.

2 Elevate burned arms or legs higher than the heart. Treat for **SHOCK,** pages 188-189.

CHEST INJURIES: CRUSHED CHEST

CHEST INJURIES: CRUSHED CHEST

134

CHEST INJURIES: CRUSHED CHEST

IMPORTANT: Seek medical aid immediately.
Observe for **SHOCK,** pages 188-189.

SYMPTOMS: Many broken ribs. The chest may collapse rather than expand when the child tries to inhale.

1 Open the child's air passage by gently tipping back his head.

2A If the injury is only on one side, turn the injured side down if possible, and try to make the child comfortable.

2B If the injury is in the center of the chest or on both sides or if he has trouble breathing, prop him up in a comfortable position.

3 If necessary, begin rescue breathing immediately; see **BREATHING: ARTIFICIAL RESPIRATION,** pages 124-127. Watch his pulse closely. If it stops, treat for **HEART FAILURE** immediately; see pages 170-173.

135

CHEST INJURIES: OPEN CHEST WOUNDS

SANDWICH BAGS

1

2

3

4

136

IMPORTANT: Seek medical aid immediately.

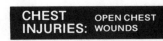

1 Seal the wound immediately with a nonporous dressing—plastic tape, aluminum foil, etc.

2 Tape the seal in place.

3 Turn the child onto the injured side, and keep his air passage open. Treat for **SHOCK,** pages 188-189.

4 If the child worsens shortly after the wound is sealed, his lung may have collapsed, in which case remove the seal immediately and listen for the escape of air. Replace the seal quickly before air is sucked into the wound.

CHEST INJURIES: RIBS

1

2

3

SYMPTOMS: The child feels pain when he inhales or when the rib area is touched.

CHEST INJURIES: RIBS

1 Place the arm on the injured side across the child's chest.

2 Bind the arm in place with bandages. **Do not** tie too tightly.

3 For support, tie another bandage along the angle of the arm. **Seek medical aid.**

CHOKING

IMPORTANT: Do not interfere with the child's own efforts to free the obstruction if he can breathe, speak or cough. If he can't, do the following:

1A If the child is standing, support his chest with one hand, and with the heel of the other, give him 4 rapid forceful blows between the shoulder blades.

1B If he is lying down, place your knee against his chest for support and administer blows.

1C Place an infant or young child face down over your forearm and administer blows.

2 If the obstruction is not cleared: Place your arms around the child, with the thumb side of your fist against his stomach between the navel and the rib cage. Grasp your fist with your other hand and make 4 quick upward thrusts at the exact spot shown. Adjust the force of your thrust to the child's size. Repeat if necessary. Watch breathing closely. If necessary, see **BREATHING: ARTIFICIAL RESPIRATION,** pages 124-127.

1

2

142

CONVULSIONS & SEIZURES

IMPORTANT: Do not give the child anything to drink during the convulsion. Tell your doctor about all convulsive seizures, no matter how brief.

SYMPTOMS: Falling. Frothing at the mouth. Stiffening of the body. Jerky, uncontrollable movements. Unconsciousness.

1 Clear the area of hard or sharp objects that might cause harm. Try to loosen tight clothing, but **do not** restrain the child.

2 When the convulsion subsides, turn the child onto her left side. Watch breathing closely. If necessary, see **BREATHING: ARTIFICIAL RESPIRATION,** pages 124-127.

DROWNING: WATER RESCUE

DROWNING: WATER RESCUE

144

IMPORTANT: Send for help immediately.
Do not swim to the child unless you cannot use reaching assists from land and it is a matter of life or death.

1A Try to reach the child from land with a hand, leg, clothing, pole, rope, etc. Throw him a buoy, board, or anything that floats. Always hold onto something with your other hand. **Do not** let the child grab you.

DROWNING: WATER RESCUE

1B If he is too far to reach, wade in closer with reaching assists.

1C If you must swim to him, keep watching him or the spot you saw him last. Bring something for the child to hold onto and pull him to shore.

2 If necessary, begin rescue breathing immediately, even before leaving the water. See **BREATHING: ARTIFICIAL RESPIRATION,** pages 124-127.

DROWNING: ICE RESCUE

DROWNING: ICE RESCUE

IMPORTANT: Send for help immediately.
Do not walk near the open ice.
Tell the child not to try to climb out but to slide his arms onto the ice and hold on until you reach him.
When safely back on firm footing, watch the child's breathing closely. If necessary, begin rescue breathing immediately. See **BREATHING: ARTIFICIAL RESPIRATION,** pages 124-127.
Observe for **SHOCK,** pages 188-189.

DROWNING: ICE RESCUE

1A Try to reach the child from land with a hand, leg, clothing, rope, ladder, sled, board, etc. Tell him to hold onto the reaching assist and slide—**not** walk upright—back to firm footing.

1B If necessary, form a human chain. Each person lies spread-eagled on the ice, holding the ankles of the person in front of him.

2 Warm the child with blankets, etc., and give him a warm, sweetened drink. If necessary, see **FROSTBITE & COLD EXPOSURE,** pages 158-161.

EAR INJURIES:

FOREIGN OBJECTS

CUTS

EAR INJURIES:

IMPORTANT: If the **ear is severed,** pack it in a cold, wet dressing and take to the hospital with the child. See **AMPUTATIONS,** pages 110-111. Blood or clear fluid coming from the ear suggests a serious **HEAD INJURY;** see pages 162-163.
For a **perforated eardrum,** place a small ball of cotton loosely in the outer ear canal and **seek medical aid immediately.**

FOREIGN OBJECTS

1 Turn the child's head onto the injured side and seek medical aid immediately. **Do not** try to remove the object yourself.

CUTS

1 Control the bleeding by pressing gauze or a clean cloth directly over the wound and elevating the child's head. Apply a wide bandage to sustain the pressure.

ELECTRIC SHOCK

1A

FUSE

1B

1C

2

150

IMPORTANT: Do not touch the child directly while he remains in contact with the current.

1A Try to turn off the current by removing the fuse or unplugging the electrical cord from the outlet.

1B If that isn't possible, stand on something dry —a blanket, rubber mat, newspapers, etc.— and push the child away with a dry board or pole.

1C Or pull the child away with a dry rope looped over the foot or arm.

2 If necessary, begin rescue breathing immediately; see **BREATHING: ARTIFICIAL RESPIRATION,** pages 124-127.
Treat for **SHOCK,** pages 188-189, and **BURNS,** pages 130-131.

EYE INJURIES: FOREIGN OBJECTS & CHEMICALS

FOREIGN OBJECTS: UPPER EYELID

CHEMICALS IN THE EYE

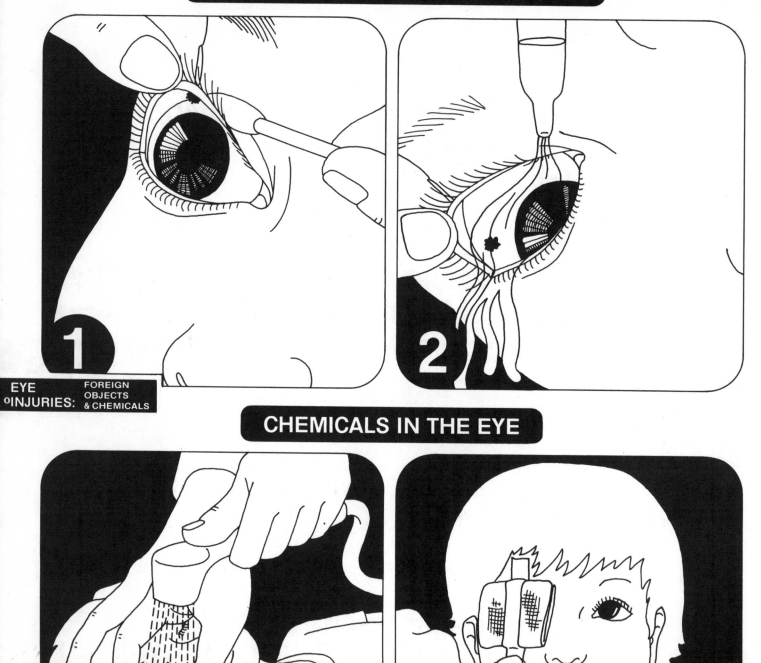

EYE INJURIES: FOREIGN OBJECTS & CHEMICALS

NOTE: Foreign objects in the lower eyelid can usually be removed with a clean handkerchief or cloth.

FOREIGN OBJECTS: UPPER EYELID

1 Clasp the upper lash between your thumb and forefinger, and fold it back over an applicator swab.

2 Have the child look down to expose the upper surface of the eyeball, then wash out the eye with water, letting the water drain down and away from the eye.

CHEMICALS IN THE EYE

1 Holding the eyelid open, flush the eye immediately in gently running water for at least 5 minutes. **Do not** let the water run into the other eye.

2 Apply gauze or a clean cloth, and hold it in place with a loosely fastened bandage. **Seek medical aid.**

EYE INJURIES: EYELID, EYEBALL & IMPALED OBJECTS

LACERATED EYEBALL

IMPALED OBJECTS

EYE INJURIES:

IMPORTANT: Seek medical aid immediately.
Do not wash out the eye.
If you must move the child, use a stretcher. See **TRANSPORTING THE INJURED,** page 198.

NOTE: Control the bleeding of a **lacerated eyelid** with a pressure dressing or direct pressure against the lid and bone.

LACERATED EYEBALL

1 Cover both eyes loosely with gauze or a clean cloth. **Do not** apply pressure. Secure the child's hands so he cannot touch his eyes.

IMPALED OBJECTS

EYE INJURIES: EYELID, EYEBALL & IMPALED OBJECTS

1 **Do not** try to remove. Cut a large hole in the center of a thick dressing, and apply the dressing carefully so it doesn't touch the eye or object.

2 Place a paper cup or cone over the eye. **Do not** touch the eye itself.

3 Secure the cup in place with a gauze or clean cloth dressing. Bandage both eyes to prevent movement in the injured eye.

IMPORTANT: Call your doctor for any fever.
Do not use medication, enemas, or alcohol or ice water rubs unless your doctor so advises.
If the fever is 103° F. (39.4° C.) or higher and you can't reach your doctor, begin gently cooling the child as described below.

1 Undress the child in a cool (**not cold**) well ventilated room. Avoid drafts and chilling.

2 Place the child in a partially filled tub of lukewarm water, keeping most of his body exposed to the air.

FEVER

3 Sponge his entire body with light, brisk strokes for 15 to 20 minutes. (If a tub isn't handy, use a sponge bath.)

4 Dry the child vigorously. Watch his temperature closely, and repeat cooling if necessary.

FROSTBITE

IMPORTANT: Do not rub or massage affected areas.

Do not apply hot water or strong heat.

Do not break blisters.

Do not give the child anything alcoholic to drink.

1 Warm the frozen parts against the body.

2 Take the child indoors. Remove clothing restricting circulation. Immerse frozen parts in warm (**not hot**) water, or cover lightly with warm towels or blankets. Discontinue warming when parts become flushed. Raise and lower affected limbs to stimulate circulation. Give the child warm soup, tea, etc.

FROSTBITE

3 Keep affected toes or fingers separated with dry gauze or clean cloth.

4 If the child must go to the hospital, bandage affected areas.

COLD EXPOSURE: HYPOTHERMIA

COLD EXPOSURE: HYPOTHERMIA

IMPORTANT: Hypothermia is the severe lowering of the temperature of the core of the body. It is usually caused by cold or cool temperatures, wind, immersion in water or wet clothing. It can become extremely serious in a matter of minutes.
Do not let the child fall asleep.
Watch breathing closely. If it stops, see **BREATHING: ARTIFICIAL RESPIRATION,** pages 124-127.

SYMPTOMS: Persistent or violent shivering. Slow or slurred speech. Loss of control of the hands. Stumbling. Exhaustion. Drowsiness. The child may not acknowledge symptoms.

1 Get the child out of the wind and cold to a warm place.

2 Remove his clothing and put him in a bed or sleeping bag. Warm his body with your own through skin-to-skin COLD EXPOSURE: HYPOTHERMIA contact. If possible, maximize the warming process with another person.

3 If he is conscious, give him warm sweet drinks or soup.

HEAD
INJURIES: CLOSED HEAD
INJURIES

IMPORTANT: Head injuries may be more severe than they seem. To be safe, **call your doctor immediately.**

Watch breathing closely. If necessary, see **BREATHING: ARTIFICIAL RESPIRATION,** pages 124-127.

Do not move the child unless absolutely necessary. If you must move him, see **TRANSPORTING THE INJURED,** pages 196-199. If the child is unconscious, assume there is a neck injury. See **BACK & NECK INJURIES,** pages 86-87. Note how long he remains unconscious.

Observe for **SHOCK,** pages 188-189.

SYMPTOMS OF SERIOUS HEAD INJURIES: Unconsciousness. Difficulty breathing. Vomiting. Convulsions. Clear fluid or blood running from ears, nose or mouth. Paralysis of any part of the body. Loss of bowel or bladder control. Unequal pupils. Skull deformity.

1 Keep the child lying down. If there is no sign of neck injury, place a pillow, jacket, etc. under both his head and his shoulders, **not** his head alone.

HEAD INJURIES: CLOSED HEAD INJURIES

2 Turn his head to one side so fluids may drain from his mouth.

HEAD INJURIES: OPEN HEAD INJURIES

164

IMPORTANT: Seek medical aid immediately.
Do not attempt to clean deep scalp wounds of foreign matter. For serious head wounds, treat for **SHOCK,** pages 188-189.

1 Control bleeding by raising the child's head and shoulders higher than her heart. **Do not** bend her neck.

2 Further control bleeding by lightly pressing gauze or a clean cloth on the wound. Avoid heavy pressure.

3 Clean minor head wounds carefully.

4 When bleeding is under control, bandage the dressing in place.

HEAD INJURIES: IMPALED OBJECTS: SKULL & CHEEK

HEAD INJURIES: IMPALED OBJECTS: SKULL & CHEEK

IMPORTANT: Seek medical aid immediately.

NOTE: Do not remove an impaled object from the skull. See **IMPALED OBJECTS,** pages 106-107.

IMPALED OBJECTS: CHEEK

1 Try to remove the object by pulling it carefully from the angle it entered the cheek. **Do not force. (For an impaled fishhook, seek medical aid.)**

2 Control the bleeding by packing the inside of the cheek with gauze or a clean cloth.

HEAD INJURIES: IMPALED OBJECTS: SKULL & CHEEK

HEAD INJURIES: FACE & JAW

HEAD INJURIES: FACE & JAW

168

HEAD INJURIES:

IMPORTANT: Seek medical aid.
Remove all broken teeth and foreign matter from the child's mouth. Save the teeth for possible replanting.
Observe for **SHOCK,** pages 188-189.

1A Raise the head higher than the heart, and control bleeding through direct pressure with gauze or a clean cloth.

1B If necessary, also press the indicated pressure point until bleeding is brought under control.

2 Apply a clean dressing or cloth, and hold it in place with a bandage.

3 For a jaw injury, support the lowered jaw in the position found with a wide bandage. If the child vomits or continues to bleed, remove the bandage, then replace when under control. Also see **CLOSED HEAD INJURIES,** pages 162-163.

HEART FAILURE:

1

HEART FAILURE: INFANT & SMALL CHILD

2

3

170

IMPORTANT: Send for an ambulance and oxygen immediately. Waste no time, but be certain all symptoms are present before you begin first aid. To check unconsciousness, call the child loudly and pinch him on the shoulder.

SYMPTOMS: Unconsciousness. No breathing. No pulse just below the left nipple.

1 Place the child on his back on a firm surface and gently tip back his head. Look and listen for air leaving his lungs. If breathing does not resume, put your open mouth over his nose and mouth, forming an airtight seal and give 4 quick, gentle puffs of air. Re-check all symptoms. If the pulse has started, see **BREATHING: ARTIFICIAL RESPIRATION,** pages 124-125. If the pulse has not started, then:

2 Place the tips of your index and middle fingers on the exact spot shown. (**Do not** press the lower end of the sternum.) Support the child's back with your other hand.

3 Make short, quick thrusts down toward the backbone about 1/2 to 3/4 of an inch, 100 times a minute. After every 5 compressions, breathe into the child's mouth (using short gentle puffs of air) as your fingertips begin to rise. If breathing seems blocked, see **CHOKING,** pages 140-141, then resume treatment. (**Do not** remove fingertips between compressions.) Discontinue compressions when the heartbeat is restored; continue rescue breathing until the child breathes spontaneously.

IMPORTANT: Send for an ambulance and oxygen immediately. If possible, have one person perform rescue breathing and another administer heart compressions. If alone, you will have to do both simultaneously. **Waste no time, but be certain all symptoms are present before you begin first aid.** To check unconsciousness, call the child loudly and pinch her on the shoulder.

SYMPTOMS: Unconsciousness. No breathing. No pulse at the large artery of the neck.

1 Place the child on her back on a firm surface and gently tip back her head. Look and listen for air leaving her lungs. If breathing does not resume, open her mouth and pinch her nose closed. Put your open mouth over her mouth, forming an airtight seal, and give 4 quick, gentle breaths. Re-check all symptoms. If the pulse has started, see **BREATHING: ARTIFICIAL RESPIRATION,** pages 126-127. If the pulse has not started, then:

2 Place the heel of one hand about 2 finger widths above the tip of the sternum. (**Do not** press the tip.)

3 Make short, quick thrusts down toward the backbone about 3/4 to 1-1/2 inches, 80 times a minute. After every 5 compressions, breathe gently into the child's mouth as the heel of your hand begins to rise. If breathing seems blocked, see **CHOKING,** pages 140-141, then resume treatment. (**Do not** remove your hand between compressions.) Discontinue compressions when the heartbeat is restored; continue rescue breathing until the child breathes spontaneously.

HEART ATTACK

HEART ATTACK

IMPORTANT: Send for an ambulance and oxygen immediately.

SYMPTOMS: Persistent pain at the center of the chest, which may radiate to the shoulders, arms, neck or jaw. Extreme shortness of breath. Anxiety. Pale or bluish lips, skin and fingernails.

1A Sit the child up and loosen his clothing. Provide good ventilation but avoid chilling.

1B If unconscious, place him on his back and tilt his head back to open his air passage. Check his breathing closely.

2 If necessary, start rescue breathing immediately. See **BREATHING: ARTIFICIAL RESPIRATION,** pages 124-127. If breathing does not resume and there is no pulse, see **HEART FAILURE,** pages 170-173.

MOUTH INJURIES: GUMS, PALATE, TEETH, LIPS & TONGUE

GUMS & PALATE

TEETH

LIPS

TONGUE

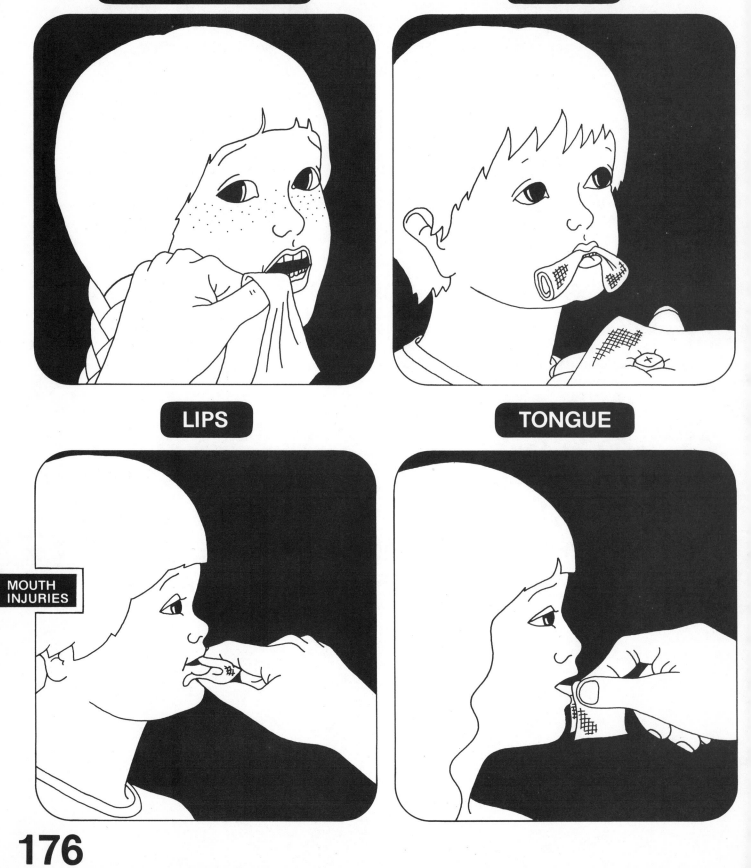

MOUTH INJURIES:

IMPORTANT: Check if there are more serious injuries to the head or neck. If necessary, see **HEAD INJURIES,** pages 162-163, and **BACK & NECK INJURIES,** pages 86-87.

Clear the mouth of broken teeth. Bring them to the doctor or dentist for possible replanting.

Lean the child slightly forward so he does not inhale blood.

GUMS & PALATE

Control bleeding by direct pressure.

TEETH

Control bleeding by direct pressure on the tooth socket. Have the child bite down firmly to hold the dressing in place.

LIPS

Control bleeding by pressing both sides of the wound.

TONGUE

Control bleeding by pressing both sides of the tongue. For more severe bleeding, gently pull the tongue and hold it for about 5 minutes.

NOSE INJURIES: FOREIGN OBJECTS, NOSE BLEED & BROKEN NOSE

NOSE BLEED

BROKEN NOSE

178

NOTE: If a **foreign object** cannot be blown out easily with both nostrils open, **do not** try to remove it. **See your doctor immediately.**

NOSE BLEED

1 Gently pinch the lower, soft part of the nose for about 5 minutes and apply cold compresses.

2 If bleeding persists, pack the nostril with absorbent cotton or gauze, then pinch the nose closed for about 10 minutes.

BROKEN NOSE

1 Control the bleeding as for **NOSE BLEED.** Tilt the child's head back slightly, and gently press cold compresses over the nose. **Do not** splint. **Seek medical aid.**

NOSE
INJURIES

179

IMPORTANT: Call your local Poison Control Center immediately. Also seek medical aid. Save the poison container and a sample of the vomit.

Watch breathing closely. If necessary, see **BREATHING: ARTIFICIAL RESPIRATION,** pages 124-127.

Do not give the child anything to drink if he is unconscious.

If you cannot reach a Poison Control Center or doctor:
- Find the poison swallowed on the list below.
- Follow the corresponding treatment on the opposite page.
- If you don't know what was swallowed, follow treatment Ⓐ. If there are no burns around the mouth, also have the child drink 5 or 6 heaping teaspoons of activated charcoal mixed in a glass of water.

Acetone Ⓑ
After Shave Lotion Ⓑ
Alcohol Ⓑ
Antifreeze Ⓑ
Arsenic Ⓑ
Battery Acid Ⓐ
Benzine Ⓑ
Bichloride of Mercury Ⓑ
Bleach Ⓑ
Body Conditioner Ⓑ
Boric Acid Ⓑ
Brush Cleaner Ⓐ
Camphor Ⓑ
Carbon Tetrachloride Ⓑ
Charcoal Lighter Ⓐ
Chlordane Ⓑ
Cologne Ⓑ
Corn Remover Ⓐ
Cosmetics Ⓑ

DDT Ⓑ
Deodorant Ⓑ
Detergent Ⓑ
Dishwasher Granules Ⓐ
Drain Cleaner Ⓐ
Fabric Softeners Ⓑ

Fingernail Polish & Remover Ⓑ
Fireworks Ⓑ
Floor Polish Ⓐ
Fluoride Ⓑ
Furniture Polish Ⓐ
Gasoline Ⓐ
Grease Remover Ⓐ
Gun Cleaner Ⓐ
Hair Dye Ⓑ
Hair Permanent Neutralizer Ⓑ
Hair Preparations Ⓑ
Hydrogen Peroxide Ⓑ
Indelible Markers Ⓑ
Ink (Green & Purple) Ⓑ
Insecticides Ⓑ
Iodine Ⓑ
Kerosene Ⓐ
Lacquer Thinner Ⓐ
Liniment Ⓑ
Lye Ⓐ
Matches (more than 20 wooden matches or 2 match books) Ⓑ
Mercury Salts Ⓑ
Metal Cleaner Ⓐ

Mothballs, Flakes or Cakes Ⓑ
Naphtha Ⓐ
Oil of Wintergreen Ⓑ
Oven Cleaner Ⓐ
Paint (Lead) Ⓑ
Paint Thinner Ⓐ
Perfume Ⓑ
Pesticides Ⓑ
Pine Oil Ⓑ
Quicklime Ⓐ
Rat or Mouse Poison Ⓑ
Roach Poison Ⓑ
Shoe Polish Ⓐ
Strychnine Ⓑ
Suntan Preparations Ⓑ
Toilet Bowl Cleaner Ⓐ
Turpentine Ⓑ
Typewriter Cleaner Ⓐ
Wart Remover Ⓐ
Washing Soda Ⓐ
Wax (Floor or Furniture) Ⓐ
Weed Killer Ⓑ
Wick Deodorizer Ⓑ
Wood Preservative Ⓐ
Zinc Compounds Ⓐ

(A) FOR ACID, ALKALI & PETROLEUM POISONING

IMPORTANT: Do not induce vomiting.

SYMPTOMS OF ACID & ALKALI POISONING: Burns around the mouth, lips and tongue. Burning sensations in the mouth, throat and stomach. Cramps. Disorientation. Bloody diarrhea.

SYMPTOMS OF PETROLEUM POISONING: Burning irritation. Coughing. Coma.

1 If the child is conscious, give him 1 or 2 glasses of milk to dilute the poison. (If milk isn't available, use water.)

2 Loosen tight clothing and treat for **SHOCK,** pages 188-189.

(B) FOR OTHER POISONING

IMPORTANT: Do not wait for symptoms to develop.

SYMPTOMS: May include nausea, dizziness, drowsiness, slurred speech, lack of coordination, cold clammy skin, thirst, convulsions, coma.

1 If the child is conscious, give him 1 or 2 glasses of milk to dilute the poison. (If milk isn't available, use water.)

2 Induce vomiting by giving him 1 tablespoon of syrup of ipecac. Keep the child moving. If he doesn't vomit within 15 minutes, give him a second tablespoon, but **do not** repeat a third time. If he still hasn't vomited within the next 30 minutes, you **must** induce vomiting by placing your finger or a spoon on the back of his tongue. **Use this method immediately if ipecac isn't available.**

3 When he starts to vomit, make sure his head is between his legs.

4 When he has finished vomiting, give him 5 or 6 heaping teaspoons of activated charcoal mixed in a glass of water.

5 Loosen tight clothing and treat for **SHOCK,** pages 188-189.

IMPORTANT: Seek medical aid and oxygen immediately. Also call your local Poison Control Center.
Watch breathing closely. If necessary, see **BREATHING: ARTIFICIAL RESPIRATION,** pages 124-127.

SYMPTOMS: Irritated eyes, nose, throat or lungs. Coughing. Headache. Shortness of breath. Nausea. Dizziness. Convulsions. Unconsciousness. Caused by auto exhaust or chemical fumes from paints, solvents and industrial gases.

1 Remove the child from the source of the poison.

2 Loosen tight clothing and treat for **SHOCK,** pages 188-189. Keep him from becoming chilled. If his skin is affected by chemical vapor or mist, see **BURNS: CHEMICAL,** pages 128-129.

POISON IVY

POISON OAK

POISON SUMAC

1

2

IMPORTANT: Seek medical aid if there is a severe reaction or the child is highly allergic.

Watch breathing closely. If necessary, see **BREATHING: ARTIFICIAL RESPIRATION,** pages 124-127.

SYMPTOMS: Burning and itching. Rash. Blisters. Swelling. Headache. Fever.

1 Remove contaminated clothing. Wash all affected areas thoroughly with soap and water, then apply rubbing alcohol.

2 Apply calamine lotion to ease the itching.

POISONING:

IMPORTANT: Call your local Poison Control Center immediately. Also seek medical aid.

Watch breathing closely. If necessary, see **BREATHING: ARTIFICIAL RESPIRATION,** pages 124-127.

Do not give the child anything to drink if he is unconscious.

If you cannot reach a Poison Control Center or doctor, see SWALLOWED POISONS, pages 180-181 and follow treatment Ⓑ.

BANEBERRY

SYMPTOMS: Dizziness. Cramps. Vomiting. Headache. Delirium.

BITTERSWEET

SYMPTOMS: Burning sensation in the throat. Nausea. Dizziness. Dilated pupils. Weakness. Convulsions.

CASTOR BEAN

SYMPTOMS: Burning sensations in the mouth and throat. Nausea. Vomiting. Cramps. Stupor. Convulsions.

DAPHNE

SYMPTOMS: Burning sensations in the mouth, throat and stomach. Cramps.

FOXGLOVE

SYMPTOMS: Nausea. Upset stomach. Dizziness. Disorientation.

JIMSON WEED

SYMPTOMS: Extreme thirst. Impaired vision. Rapid heartbeat. Dilated pupils. Delirium. Coma.

LARKSPUR (DELPHINIUM)

SYMPTOMS: Tingling in the mouth. Upset stomach. Anxiety. Severe depression.

LILY-OF-THE-VALLEY

SYMPTOMS: Upset stomach. Dizziness. Vomiting. Disorientation.

MONKSHOOD

SYMPTOMS: Tingling or numbness of the lips and tongue. Excessive salivating. Dizziness. Nausea. Vomiting. Dimmed vision.

NIGHTSHADE

SYMPTOMS: Thirst. Upset stomach. Numbness. Rapid heartbeat.

POISON HEMLOCK

SYMPTOMS: Burning sensations in the mouth and throat. Weakness. Paralysis of the arms and chest. Stupor.

POKEWEED

SYMPTOMS: Burning sensations in the mouth and throat. Nausea. Cramps. Upset stomach. Vomiting. Drowsiness. Impaired vision.

WATER HEMLOCK

SYMPTOMS: Excessive salivating. Foaming at the mouth. Stomach pain. Frenzy. Shivering. Irregular breathing. Delirium. Violent convulsions.

YEW

SYMPTOMS: Nausea. Stomach pain. Vomiting. Shivering. Difficulty breathing. Diarrhea.

1

2A

2B

SHOCK

3

IMPORTANT: Always treat a seriously injured child for shock.
Do not give the child anything to drink.
Do not overheat.
Seek medical aid immediately.

SYMPTOMS: Pale, cold, clammy skin, mottled in color. Breathing is weak and shallow or deep but irregular. Apathy. Nausea.

1 Lay the child down. Place a blanket under him if he is cold or damp, but **do not** move him if his back or neck is injured.

2A If his head is injured or he has trouble breathing, elevate his neck and shoulders.

2B Otherwise, elevate his legs about 8 to 12 inches, unless that causes pain.

3 Cover the child lightly with a blanket.

SPRAINS & STRAINS

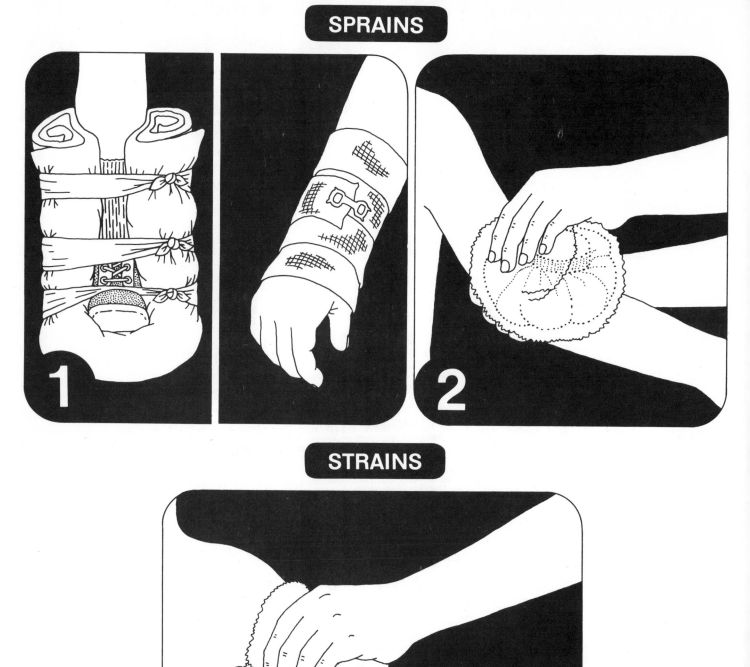

SPRAINS

1

2

STRAINS

1

SPRAINS & STRAINS

IMPORTANT: Keep the child off the injured parts.
Do not pack in ice or immerse in ice water.

SPRAINS

SYMPTOMS: Pain, rapid swelling, tenderness and discoloration of the soft tissue surrounding a joint.

1 Immobilize the injured area with a blanket, splint, pillow, elasticized bandage, etc. **Do not** bandage too tightly; sprains swell.

2 To minimize swelling, elevate sprained elbows, knees or ankles. Apply cold, wet compresses or an ice bag covered with a towel.

STRAINS

SYMPTOMS: Pain caused by stretched or pulled muscles.

1 Apply warm, wet compresses and rest the injured part.

IMPORTANT: Do not give the child anything to drink.
If breathing becomes difficult, elevate the head and shoulders.
For **IMPALED OBJECTS,** see pages 106-107.
Seek medical aid immediately.

1 Relax the stomach muscles by placing the child on his back with a pillow or blanket under his knees.

2 Control bleeding by applying direct pressure on the wound with gauze or a clean cloth.

3 Bandage the dressing firmly in place.

4 If organs or intestines protrude, **do not** attempt to replace them. Cover the area with a clean dressing dampened with sterile or cooled boiled water. Bandage in place firmly but not too tightly. Treat for **SHOCK,** pages 188-189.

SUNSTROKE & HEAT EXHAUSTION

SUNSTROKE

1A

1B

HEAT EXHAUSTION

1

2

SUNSTROKE & HEAT EXHAUSTION

SUNSTROKE

IMPORTANT: Seek medical aid immediately.
Act quickly. Body temperature must be lowered at once. Watch temperature closely. Repeat first-aid treatment if temperature rises. **Do not** give stimulants.

SYMPTOMS: Body temperature is extremely high. Skin is flushed and dry. No sweating.

1A Place the child in a partially filled tub of cool water. Using light, brisk strokes, sponge his entire body until temperature is reduced.

1B Or take the child to a cool, well ventilated room, and wrap him in wet, cold sheets until temperature is reduced.

HEAT EXHAUSTION

SYMPTOMS: Moist skin. Cramps or muscle spasms. Body temperature is normal or subnormal.

1 Take the child to a cool, shaded, well ventilated room. Remove her clothing and have her lie down. Cool her off with fans, an air conditioner or cool, moist cloths.

2 If the child is conscious, give her sips of salt water (1 teaspoon in a glass) every few minutes for one hour. Have the child rest, then give her sweetened iced tea or iced coffee.

IMPORTANT: If the child is seriously injured, call an ambulance immediately. Do not move him unless it is a matter of life or death and no ambulance is available. It is almost always better to wait for proper equipment and expert help. If you must transport the child, get as much aid as possible.

1 Devise a stretcher out of a sturdy board, door, ironing board, etc.

2 **Do not** twist the child. Move his body as a single unit, keeping his head in line with his spinal column. On a signal from the person holding the head, roll him gently onto his side and place the stretcher next to him.

3 Roll him onto the stretcher carefully without twisting his body or head.

4 Immobilize his head with a rolled blanket or the like. (For spine injuries, also immobilize his torso.) Bind him to the stretcher with bandages, belts, etc.

IMPROVISED STRETCHERS

CHAIR CARRY

ONE-PERSON LIFT

FIREMAN & PACK-STRAP

TWO-MAN SEAT

For our free brochure of child safety products,
send your name and address to:

West Stockbridge, Massachusetts 01266